AF832542

THE POLITICS OF AIDS DENIALISM

Global Health

Series Editors: Professor Nana K. Poku, John Ferguson Professor, University of Bradford, UK and Dr Robert L. Ostergard, Assistant Professor, University of Nevada, USA and Research Fellow Centre of Democractic Performance

The benefits of globalization are potentially enormous, as a result of the increased sharing of ideas, cultures, life-saving technologies and efficient production processes. Yet globalization is under trial, partly because these benefits are not yet reaching hundreds of millions of the world's poor and partly because globalization has introduced new kinds of international problems and conflicts. Turmoil in one part of the world now spreads rapidly to others, through terrorism, armed conflict, environmental degradation or disease.

This timely series provides a robust and multi-disciplinary assessment of the asymmetrical nature of globalization. Books in the series encompass a variety of areas, including global health and the politics of governance, poverty and insecurity, gender and health and the implications of global pandemics.

Also in the series

Gender and HIV/AIDS
Critical Perspectives from the Developing World
Edited by Jelke Boesten and Nana K. Poku
ISBN 978 0 7546 7269 2

AIDS, South Africa, and the Politics of Knowledge
Jeremy R. Youde
ISBN 978 0 7546 7003 2

AIDS and Governance
Edited by Nana K. Poku, Alan Whiteside and Bjorg Sandkjaer
ISBN 978 0 7546 4579 5

The Political Economy of AIDS in Africa
Edited by Nana K. Poku and Alan Whiteside
ISBN 978 0 7546 3897 1

The Politics of AIDS Denialism
South Africa's Failure to Respond

PIETER FOURIE
Macquarie University, Australia
and
MELISSA MEYER
HIV/AIDS and the Media Project, South Africa

Routledge
Taylor & Francis Group
LONDON AND NEW YORK

First published 2010 by Ashgate Publishing

Published 2016 by Routledge
2 Park Square, Milton Park, Abingdon, Oxon OX14 4RN
711 Third Avenue, New York, NY 10017, USA

Routledge is an imprint of the Taylor & Francis Group, an informa business

Copyright © Pieter Fourie and Melissa Meyer 2010

Pieter Fourie and Melissa Meyer have asserted their right under the Copyright, Designs and Patents Act, 1988, to be identified as the authors of this work.

All rights reserved. No part of this book may be reprinted or reproduced or utilised in any form or by any electronic, mechanical, or other means, now known or hereafter invented, including photocopying and recording, or in any information storage or retrieval system, without permission in writing from the publishers.

Notice:
Product or corporate names may be trademarks or registered trademarks, and are used only for identification and explanation without intent to infringe.

British Library Cataloguing in Publication Data
Fourie, Pieter, 1972-
The politics of AIDS denialism : South Africa's failure to respond. -- (Global health)
1. AIDS (Disease)--South Africa--Epidemiology. 2. AIDS (Disease)--Government policy--South Africa--History.
3. AIDS (Disease)--Political aspects--South Africa.
4. AIDS (Disease)--Social aspects--South Africa.
I. Title II. Series III. Meyer, Melissa.
362.1'969792'00968-dc22

Library of Congress Cataloging-in-Publication Data
Fourie, Pieter, 1972-
The politics of AIDS denialism : South Africa's failure to respond / by Pieter Fourie and Melissa Meyer.
p. ; cm. -- (Global health)
Includes bibliographical references and index.
ISBN 978-1-4094-0405-7 (hbk) 1. AIDS (Disease)--Government policy--South Africa. 2. Denial (Psychology)--South Africa. I. Meyer, Melissa, 1985- II. Title. III.
Series: Global health.
[DNLM: 1. HIV Infections--South Africa. 2. Acquired Immunodeficiency Syndrome--South Africa. 3. Health Policy--South Africa. WC 503 F775p 2010]
RA643.86.S6F683 2010
362.196'979200968--dc22

2010020478

ISBN 9781409404057 (hbk)

Transferred to Digital Printing 2014

Contents

List of Figures

List of Tables

Foreword

> As Adam Smith observed, 'We desire both to be respectable and to be respected'. The power of denial is equally strong. Both tendencies encourage people to ignore the damage caused by their social actions and to develop elaborate stories justifying their privileges. Both give rise to the pride that, like fear, lies behind cultural racism. They help to explain why the adage 'men make history but do not know the history they make' is true.[1]

This year marks the start of the third decade of HIV and AIDS – three decades in which the epidemic has taken hold and three decades in which the response of both civil society and government has been marked by denial, inaction and muddled policies and responses. The South African epidemic has been one of the most studied and researched, and placed under a scrutiny as no other epidemic – on the continent or throughout the world.

What drives this fascination and frustration with the South Africa HIV and AIDS epidemics? Why is the South African epidemic and the response to it such a source of research and investigation? Is it because of the magnitude of the numbers infected and dying or because this is seen to be an exceptional epidemic, unfolding in an exceptional country. How is it possible that in 1990, HIV prevalence among antenatal clinic attendees (women 15–49 years) was less than 1 per cent and yet by 2008 it has reached 29.3 per cent?[2] What explains the response of the governments in the last two decades to this epidemic as it has unfolded or the response of the health sector, the education sector and civil society.

South Africa is still, 30 years on, experiencing one of the most serious HIV/AIDS epidemics in the world. At the same time, the country has developed one of the most serious and fascinating responses to HIV and AIDS. In many ways South Africa was expected to succeed in finding ways to combat HIV and AIDS under exceptional circumstances in much the same way that it managed to defeat apartheid under exceptional circumstances. There was something about the Rainbow Nation that captured the imagination of the world, and South Africans were expected to perform miracles in a range of social issues – housing, education, service delivery, heath care including HIV and AIDS. South Africa was expected to succeed where other countries seemed to have failed.

---

1 D. Wylie, *Starving on a Full Stomach: Hunger and the Triumph of Cultural Racism in Modern South Africa* (University Press of Virginia: Charlottesville, 2001), 240.

2 National Department of Health, *National Antenatal Sentinel HIV and Syphilis Survey*, September 2009.

South Africa and its AIDS epidemic is a bewildering mix of forward thinking progressive responses and equally bewildering inaction, stupidity and stalling. The country with one of the worst epidemics in the world has also some of the very best legislation to deal with the many complex issues the epidemic throws up. Many people are denied access to treatments through state inaction and inability to ensure adequate supplies. Many people do not have access to prevention measures that can enable them to make choices and yet South Africa has, in relation to HIV and AIDS, a very strong human rights culture. There exists an impressive range of activists who have forced changes in policy and response.

Through the years there has been the National AIDS Plan of 1994, the National Strategic Plans moving beyond 2011, which attempt to unite all government departments to act on the epidemic and to take the lead where their expertise is the most appropriate. Yet, parallel to this has been the policy to support curious theories of alternative medications, using combinations of food as treatment rather than drugs. While trying to get people to take HIV and AIDS seriously and change behaviour, calls were made against the provision of ARV treatments as being toxic and unsafe.

Alongside the legislation and the national plans there has been a continual failure to implement the plans on any sustained or effective level. There has been piecemeal success and failure but there has not been decisive leadership to make the plans a reality. Alongside the progressive laws and the various programmes have been the rumblings of discontent over the issues of human rights, over the need for confidentiality and the fact that AIDS is not a fully notifiable disease. Frustrated by the seeming lack of progress there are moves to make all people who visit public health centres the 'routine' offer of a test. This is being done, in the context of a health service that in some cases cannot sustain treatment for those who are already diagnosed.

Alongside the calls to have a South Africa united against AIDS lies the discourse of race and racism in the epidemic, the discourse about the South African epidemic fuelled and directed by the West and various donors and indeed Mbeki himself of 'African sexuality' and the ways in which calls to culture both collude with and challenge the public silences and denial.

Denial has been one of the key accusations thrown at the government and much of civil society, in workplaces and at the muted education programmes. This reflects a denial of the reality of the epidemic, a denial of the need to change sexual practices, understanding and behaviour, and a denial of just how much society and our future will be affected by HIV and AIDS. An AIDS epidemic as severe as the one damaging South African society requires that we have to imagine how this change may look and how we need to plan for it.

The denial does not lie just in the failure to develop effective government interventions, effective communication strategies, or to offer testing and treatments, care and support. Denial also lies in the failure to understand what this epidemic is doing to the fabric and the soul of our country. There is no compelling talk about the impact of AIDS on families, other than accounts of misery and despair. There is no loud call to take heed of what this epidemic is doing to young people terrified and traumatised by the deaths of their parents and relatives. There is no horror at the fact that child headed households, which have no place in a caring democracy, have been allowed to exist and there has been no public ongoing debate about how we create new families, new communities, new ways of living and debating what kind of society we would all be proud to inhabit when we have moved through this epidemic.

Faced with a crumbling health service we simply plan to make the sector which is failing in all kinds of ways to take on more responsibility with regards to HIV and AIDS. In an education system that is not serving the needs of its learners or the developmental needs of the country – educators are expected to take on social welfare functions to deal with the many social aspects of the epidemic and as more people go onto treatments there is no companion call for food security and comprehensive food support. The fact that the necessity for this kind of support may, in theory, be acknowledged and offered in some places masks the fact that too many health care professionals, too many teachers, too many communities are buckling under the impact of what they are expected to deliver – and to deliver while in many cases dealing with their own infection and suffering in their extended networks.

Failure on the part of governments over three decades to develop an innovative and effective response to HIV and AIDS and the power of denial and inaction has produced the equally serious failure to take up the challenge of how this epidemic is fundamentally changing the society in which we live – changing the very deep social, cultural, race and class foundations on which social values and cohesion can be understood or built.

The most serious failure of all perhaps, has been, the failure to take HIV and AIDS as a lens through which we can re-examine society and see through it, how we can generate new debates about society, identity, power, gender, exploitation and abuse. We have failed to see how, through understanding how and why this epidemic plays out in the way that it does, we can take old social, political, economic and cultural dilemmas and consequences and look at them in new ways and find new solutions, rather than trying to buttress and defend the existing social and cultural formations.

We have failed to develop a strong critique of the epidemic and responses to it and in doing so we have failed to offer insights into how South Africa dealing with AIDS could be transformed.

It is, of course, still possible to do this critique and to challenge some of the responses and detail their consequences. Towards achieving that, this meticulously researched book, lays a solid foundation. Through its detailed analysis of what has and has not been done and through opening the debate on denial and understanding, it opens the space for a thorough development of sustained critique and the transformation of our understanding of how our society will develop, driven by the changes that will come about socially, culturally and economically due to HIV and AIDS.

Mary Crewe
Director
Centre for the Study of AIDS, University of Pretoria

This book is dedicated to the AIDS Law Project
and the Treatment Action Campaign
A luta continua!

Preface

Fact: HIV causes AIDS.
Fact: HIV does not discriminate according to individuals' race, culture, class, sex, sexual orientation, religion, age or geography.
Fact: Anti-retroviral drugs can significantly decrease national morbidity and mortality levels in the context of mature epidemics.
Fact: The provision of these drugs at scale is less expensive than simply letting people die.
Fact: Good nutrition is essential to building and sustaining individuals' resistance to disease, but are complementary and not an alternative to the function of anti-retroviral drugs in HIV-positive individuals.

None of these statements are in any way controversial. Medical science, actuarial science and even the 'dismal' science (economics) have rendered these assertions objectively and logically uncontentious. Serious arguments that dispute these statements have long been relegated to the intellectual dustbin. Only on the fringes of the fringes – amongst the irrational, the mad, the cynical, the purposefully disingenuous, or those blindly clinging to their own pathological normative scripts – are claims that run counter to the five facts stated above still taken seriously.

However, since AIDS first made its public debut in South Africa in the early 1980s such counter-claims have found remarkable traction in that country. In particular, former South African President Thabo Mbeki's views on AIDS have led to allegations that his government was in a state of denial about the AIDS epidemic. However, the long-wave nature of the epidemic suggests that the present extent of the South African epidemic is the result of *successive* South African governments' failure to respond adequately to HIV and AIDS. If denial is at least in part to blame for recent government complacency and inaction, this suggests that denial and denialism have been recurring components of official responses to HIV and AIDS since the first two South African AIDS deaths in 1982.

This book attempts to determine the validity of claims of government denial by formulating and testing a theory of denial. This denial 'hypothesis' is first contextualised with an overview of the South African epidemic as well as a review of allegations of government denial. London School of Economics and Political Science (LSE) scholar Stanley Cohen's typology of official denial is then applied to South African official rhetoric to determine whether instances of government denial have been significant as well as frequent enough to warrant claims of continual official denial. This reveals possible political factors that may motivate policy makers to resort to official denial.

The book concludes with a judgment regarding the allegations contained in this theory of denial. However, this is done within the broader notion that denial is inherently vague and couched in language (rarely in writing) and therefore difficult to test with certainty. The real value of the book lies in the insights gained into the complex politics of denial – these lessons apply to AIDS in South Africa, but also to instances of official denial about other issues, and elsewhere.

This book goes beyond existing texts regarding the South African AIDS epidemic. Very recent books as well as other publications on AIDS in South Africa over the last decade have by and large focused on the Mbeki government's quixotic AIDS policy response. This book is different in that it hopes to (1) provide a serious, comprehensive analysis of AIDS denial and denialism *per se*, and (2) then applies it not only to the Mbeki administration, but to the apartheid and Mandela governments as well.

The last point is so important that we would like to paraphrase it: this book is not about Thabo Mbeki. Or rather, this book is not an enumeration of, and an attack on, the Mbeki government's bad AIDS governance. Instead, we proffer an analytical lens or prism through which all political denial can be viewed, and we apply this perspective to not only Mbeki, but to all South African administrations who had to govern in a time of AIDS.

There are a number of institutions and individuals without whom this book would not have been possible. Rory Ryan and the Faculty of Humanities at the University of Johannesburg provided the space for both of us to pursue our individual research during our postgraduate studies. In particular, Deon Geldenhuys and Albert Venter of UJ's Department of Politics were real mentors.

Melissa Meyer would like to thank the following individuals: Ben Osborn, my best friend and greatest critic; my brother Udo, who will always make me laugh; my family back 'home' in Namibia: Gert, Martie and Carola; the Osborn family for their quiet and unwavering support; Christin English, without whom I never would have survived university; Arina Rademeyer and Elena Pellissier, who helped me build a home away from home; Ntokozo Vilakazi – cherished friend and respected 'rival'; old friends: Philipp Schier, Ettienne Bingham and De Wet Mostert; Jos Slabbert who helped me discover the idea-building power of words and Des and Anneli Erasmus, who coached me into a passion for journalism.

Pieter Fourie would like to thank the following: Rietjie Fourie, for always believing and enthusing; and then thank you also to Colleen O'Manique, Diana Perche, Anita Visser, Suzanne and Victoria Graham, Liani Lochner, Bonnie Skinner, Henning and Karin Snyman, Leon Hartwell, Maxi Schoeman, Zani Naudé, Ria Schoeman, Debbie Mathew, Tony Barnett, Nana Poku, Alan Whiteside and Mary Crewe, who always encouraged, and who made me believe that the topic is worthwhile.

We thank Stanley Cohen and Colleen O'Manique for their reflections on earlier drafts of this document, as well as the anonymous reviewers, whose comments were essential in the framing of the final text.

And last but not least, we are most grateful to Ashgate's editorial team – your good humour, flexible deadlines (!), enthusiasm for the topic, incredible focus and meticulous collaboration made it all possible, and remarkably painless.

Pieter Fourie and Melissa Meyer

List of Abbreviations

ACT UP	AIDS Coalition to Unleash Power
AIDS	Acquired Immunodeficiency Syndrome
ANC	African National Congress
ARV	Anti-retroviral
ATIC	AIDS Training and Information Centre
AVRU	AIDS Virus Research Unit
AZT	Azidothymidine
CIA	Central Intelligence Agency
COSATU	Congress of South African Trade Unions
GAAP	Government AIDS Action Plan
GEAR	Growth, Employment and Redistribution
GPA	Global Programme on AIDS
GRID	Gay Related Immunodeficiency Syndrome
HAART	Highly Active Anti-retroviral Therapy
HIV	Human Immunodeficiency Virus
IDC	Interdepartmental Committee on AIDS
IMF	International Monetary Fund
KS	Kaposi's Sarcoma
MCC	Medicines Control Council
MinMEC	Ministerial meeting of the MEC
MRC	Medical Research Council
MTCT	Mother-to-Child Transmission
MTCTP	Mother-to-Child Transmission Prevention
NACOSA	National AIDS Convention Of South Africa
NAP	National AIDS Plan
NAPWA	National Association of People Living with HIV and AIDS
NARP	National AIDS Research Programme
NEPAD	New Partnership for Africa's Development
NGO	Non-governmental organisation

NP	National Party
NSP	National Strategic Plan
PAC	Provincial AIDS Council
PCP	*pneumocystiscarinii pneumonia*
PEP	Post-exposure Prophylactic
PHRC	Provincial Heads of Health
PhrMA	Pharmaceutical Manufacturers' Association
PWA	Persons living With AIDS
RDP	Reconstruction and Development Programme
SANAC	South African National AIDS Council
SSA	Sub-Saharan Africa
STD	Sexually Transmitted Disease
STI	Sexually Transmitted Infection
TAC	Treatment Action Campaign
UN	United Nations
UNAIDS	Joint United Nations Programme on HIV and AIDS
UNDP	United Nations Development Programme
VCT	Voluntary Counselling and Testing
WHO	World Health Organisation

Chapter 1
Introduction

Thabo Mbeki's controversial views on AIDS and his two governments' objections to, and foot dragging on, treatment rollout have rendered him infamous amongst the local and global AIDS community, scientists and most of South African civil society. Amidst all the media and public relations furore, the blame for the severity of South Africa's AIDS epidemic has almost exclusively been allocated to Mbeki, his Health Minister, Manto Tshabalala-Msimang, and their denialist attitude.

But matters of blame and denial are not that easily resolved when relating to the AIDS epidemic. Firstly, this has to do with the long-wave nature of the epidemic. Its slow, creeping onset means that HIV and AIDS have become a living reality, unlike most other disasters that tend to strike suddenly, elicit shock and necessitate urgent action. Secondly, the delay between HIV infection and AIDS illness and death has implications for both the perceived severity and urgency of the epidemic as well as accountability for infections and treatment. It can take up to two Presidential terms for HIV infections to unfold into full-blown AIDS illness. The unique nature of the epidemic has serious implications for how leaders perceive their accountability and responsibility to act.

Whilst Mbeki has become a convenient scapegoat, this drawn-out nature of the epidemic necessitates a closer investigation of government response – including that of Mbeki's predecessors. Thabo Mbeki may have been at the helm of a government that refused to make lifesaving treatment available to AIDS suffers, but those who were ill and dying during Mbeki's tenure contracted HIV quite some time before he took up office. That AIDS deaths surged during this time would suggest that long before Mbeki's notorious handling of the epidemic, South African officials failed to avert the spread of HIV.

In this light the popularly held view that Mbeki's government was in a state of denial requires careful reconsideration. Taking the long-wave nature of the epidemic into account, this book argues that accusations of government denial should be reformulated to consider not only recent government (in)action, but also that of former governments that were as responsible for not adequately facing up to the realities of AIDS in South Africa.

A short history of the epidemic

The developed world's version of the story of HIV and AIDS typically begins in the early 1980s when Western doctors observed an increase in certain opportunistic illnesses amongst urban homosexual men. The pathology suggested that these patients' immune systems were compromised. In 1981 doctors in New York noted an increase in a particularly aggressive form of Kaposi's Sarcoma (KS) amongst young gay men (KS is a form of cancer that until then had been relatively benign and largely limited to older people).[1] That same year a number of cases of a rare lung infection, *pneumocystis carinii pneumonia* (PCP), were treated in California and New York.[2] Again these instances were confined to homosexual men. PCP is a condition that is common to animals like dogs, rats and sheep. Humans often carry the infection latently without falling ill. The manifestation of PCP into life-threatening pneumonia suggested to doctors that 'something was seriously wrong' (Whiteside 2006: 30).

These initial findings led to the medical community naming this new disease Gay-Related Immune Deficiency Syndrome (GRID). However, cases were soon discovered amongst haemophiliacs, Haitians and intravenous drug users (IDUs). It was not long before the name GRID was rendered redundant (Avert 2009). Thus the acronym AIDS (Acquired Immunodeficiency Syndrome) was formulated. The name 'AIDS' was first used on 27 July 1982 at a meeting in Washington, DC (Kher 2003).

Awareness and knowledge of AIDS grew rapidly. Already by 1982 a number of voluntary organisations were established in the United States (Avert 2009). By this time cases of AIDS were appearing in all developed countries (Whiteside 2006: 31). In 1983, incidents of AIDS in women suggested that the disease could be spread through heterosexual as well as homosexual intercourse.[3] That same year a team of scientists from the *Institut Pasteur* in Paris (led by French scientist Luc Monagnier) identified the cause of AIDS – the Human Immunodeficiency Virus that later became known as HIV-1.[4] A second HI virus was identified two years later, known as HIV-2. This is a much less aggressive virus that is harder to transmit, slower acting and less virulent (Whiteside 2006: 31).

By 1985 the first needle exchange programmes had been introduced to prevent HIV transmission during drug use (Avert 2009). Also in 1985, the first test for HIV was developed (Pear 1985). The following year, around 38,000 cases of AIDS had been reported to the World Health Organisation (WHO). By now developed countries were responding strongly with awareness campaigns. In February 1986 the UK held its first 'AIDS week'. That same year ACT UP (the AIDS Coalition to Unleash Power) was founded. US President Ronald Reagan also made his first major speech on AIDS and the WHO's Global Programme on AIDS (GPA)

---

1 Hymes et al. (1981) published these findings in an article titled 'Kaposi's Sarcoma in homosexual men: A report of eight cases' in *The Lancet.*

2 These PCP findings were published in the Centre for Disease Control's (CDC) Morbidity and Mortality Weekly Reports on 5 June and 4 July 1981. See MMWR (1981a) and MMWR (1981b).

3 See MMWR (1983) for epidemiologic notes and reports on the first female cases of AIDS.

4 HIV-1 was initially referred to as lymphadenopathy-associated virus, or LAV. Dr Robert Gallo of the National Cancer Institute in the US discovered the HI virus a year later and called it HTLV-III. The following year it became clear that LAV and HTLV-II were the same virus (Avert 2009).

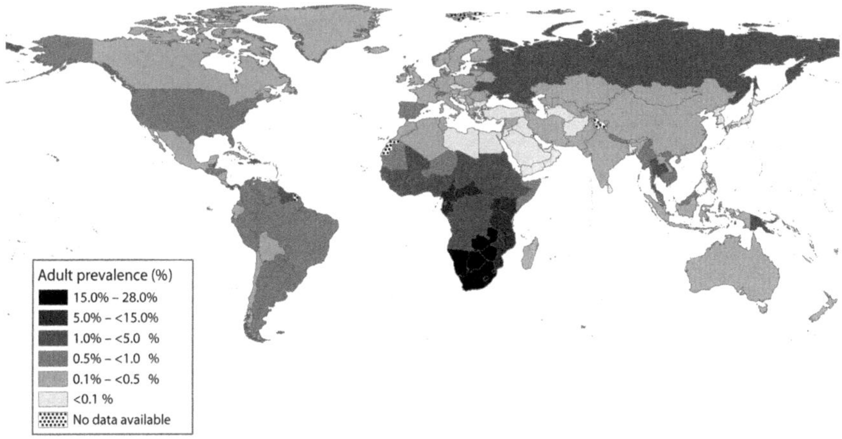

Figure 1.1 A global view of HIV infection: 2007
Source: UNAIDS (2008).

developed a Global AIDS Strategy. That same year, work on treatment for HIV and AIDS had yielded the first anti-retroviral drug, azidothymidine (AZT).[5] On 1 December 1988 the first World AIDS Day was held and the US launched a wide-reaching HIV and AIDS education campaign (Avert 2009).

The resources invested in the search for treatment continued to yield promising results into the mid-1990s. In 1994, AZT was proven to limit the risk of mother-to-child transmission (MTCT) of HIV (Connor et al. 1994). As a result infant mortality rates in developing countries declined sharply. In 1996 the first non-nucleoside reverse transcriptase inhibitor (a new treatment for HIV, Viramune, also known as Nevirapine) was released. Around that time, researchers also established the heightened efficacy of combination anti-retroviral treatment (Priority Press 1995). Consequently AIDS death tolls in the developed world declined sharply (Brown 1997).

This relatively rapid response coupled with good access to treatment have meant that in the developed world HIV and AIDS have become manageable conditions (often compared to lifestyle diseases like diabetes). As a result the epidemic in North America, Western Europe, Australia and other developed countries is quite contained, with national prevalence rates well below one per cent of the populations.

As demonstrated in Figure 1.1, by comparison, the national prevalence levels in Sub-Saharan Africa are often well in excess of five, ten or even 15 per cent (UNAIDS 2008). The total number of people living with HIV in North America, Western and

---

5 A clinical trial showed that AZT slowed down the attack of HIV (see Fischl et al. 1987).

Central Europe (2 million) is nearly equal to the amount of new infections in 2007 alone in Sub-Saharan Africa (1.9 million). It follows that for the developing world (and Africa in particular) the story of HIV and AIDS has been a very different one.

A ten-year study completed in 2005 provided conclusive evidence that HIV originated in Africa.[6] The first transfer of HIV-1 to humans is thought to have occurred around 1930.[7] Experts estimate that by the 1960s, 2,000 people in Africa were already infected. The first epidemic most likely broke out in Kinshasa in the 1970s. However, a lack of awareness of HIV and AIDS at the time led to the labelling of the illness as 'slim disease'. Unlike in developed countries, in Africa the virus was and is mostly spread heterosexually (Avert 2009).

From Kinshasa (which is often called the epicentre of the epidemic) the virus spread to Eastern Africa in the 1980s. Transmission was rapid due to a number of factors, including the migrant labour system, the low status of women, a high ratio of men in urban areas, a lack of circumcision and the prevalence of sexually transmitted infections (STIs) (Avert 2009). Around this time Uganda experienced a sudden surge in deaths caused by 'slim disease'. By the mid-1980s associations were made between slim disease and the newly discovered HI virus (Serwadda et al. 1985).

Lack of knowledge of the disease, limited access to resources and a widespread sense of fear against the backdrop of economic concerns and political instability led to an overall paralysis amongst African governments in the early stages of the epidemic. The developed world was also slow to intervene. The WHO initially argued that there were more immediate health concerns in Africa that took preference, like malaria (Avert 2009).

By the end of the 1980s, HIV and AIDS had made its way to Southern Africa. Ten years later, just as the epidemic began burgeoning in Southern Africa, prevalence rates in East Africa were slowing (Avert 2009).[8] Whilst governments as well as the international community have since been responding to the epidemic, HIV and AIDS is still worst in Africa – where it originated. Statistics from the Joint United Nations Programme on AIDS (UNAIDS) suggest that in 2007 over three quarters of the world's AIDS deaths (1.5 million) have taken place in Sub-Saharan Africa (SSA) and that over two thirds of the world's HIV cases are in SSA (22 million) (UNAIDS 2008).

In spite of the epidemic's concentration in SSA, cases of HIV and AIDS have been reported in every country, making it a global health issue. Around 33 million people were thought to be living with HIV in 2007 (UNAIDS 2008). Given its global reach this can rightfully be called a pandemic (Whiteside 2006: 28).

---

6 The study found a Simian Immunodeficiency Virus (SIV) in chimpanzee colonies in South-East Cameroon that is a viral ancestor of HIV-1 (Van Heuverswyn et al. 2006).

7 However, it has recently been suggested that HIV originated somewhere between 1884 and 1924 (Worobey et al. 2008). HIV-2 is thought to have made the transfer to humans in the 1940s, in the region of Guinea-Bissau (Lemey et al. 2003).

8 Effective intervention campaigns and behavioural change are largely credited for the decline in the East African epidemic (see Avert 2009).

HIV and AIDS in South Africa

The South African story of HIV and AIDS resounds both with the story of developed countries as well as with Africa's. The apartheid governments' rule meant that racially white areas resembled isolated strongholds of modernity in which people enjoyed the living standards, health care and technology of the developed world. Beyond the white cities and suburbs, however, poverty was rife and conditions were ideal for the rapid spread of a heterosexual epidemic. And so, in South Africa, HIV and AIDS made its onslaught on two fronts.

In 1982 two South African air stewards died of opportunistic infections associated with AIDS. Like the first cases in the US both men were homosexuals (Ras et al. 1983: 140). Soon after, HIV surfaced amongst haemophiliacs, drug users and commercial sex workers. In 1988 an increase in HIV amongst the black population was observed and it was speculated that an 'African type' heterosexual epidemic might follow (Sher 1989: 317).

It is likely that given the skewed nature of the health system under apartheid, a heterosexual epidemic was already brewing amongst the black population but that the white medical institutions were largely isolated from it. Four years later, in 1992, whilst official statistics reported only 26 AIDS deaths in the whole of South Africa, one hospital in the rural Kwa-Zulu Natal homeland alone recorded 153 AIDS deaths in the first nine months of that year (Furlong and Ball 2005: 133). Having been severely neglected under the apartheid system, the South African epidemic soon began mirroring the 'African pattern' as it evolved into a largely heterosexual epidemic.

In its severity, however, South Africa's story of HIV and AIDS is unique (see Figure 1.2). It remains the country with the largest AIDS epidemic in the world. South Africa is home to the greatest number of HIV-positive people in the world, totalling over 5.7 million in 2007 (UNAIDS 2008: 40). According to an actuarial study conducted in 2006 by Dorrington et al. (2006: 10) prevalence amongst South African men aged 30 to 34 was as high as 26.5 per cent and reached a maximum of 32.5 per cent amongst women aged 25 to 29. This means that if left untreated, at least a quarter of the backbone of South African society will fall ill and die prematurely.

In August 2009, the eminent medical journal *The Lancet* (2009) stated that, since 1994, average life expectancy in South Africa has dropped by almost 20 years, mainly because of the rise in HIV-related mortality. Average life expectancy at birth is only 50 years for men and 54 years for women, and according to the South African Institute of Race Relations' annual survey (SAIRR 2009), by 2011 life expectancy will fall to 48 years for men and 51 years for women. The *Lancet* study points out that South Africa has 0.7 per cent of the world's population, but carries 17 per cent of the global HIV burden.

The implications that an epidemic of such magnitude has for South African society are immense. AIDS deaths leave both the elderly and the young without caregivers and in so doing negate the intergenerational contract that holds parents

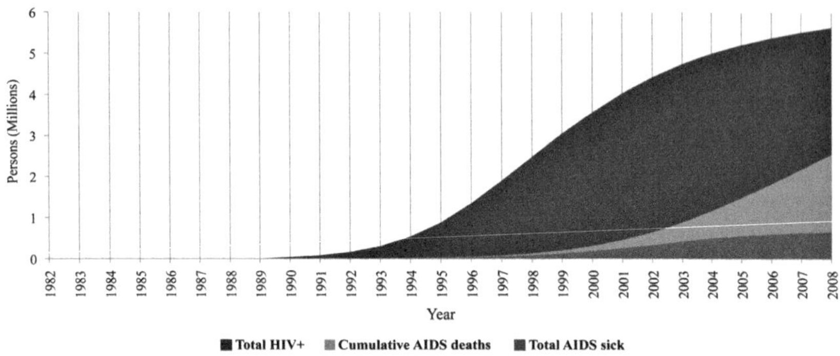

Figure 1.2 The South African AIDS epidemic

Source: Data compiled from Dorrington et al. (2006).

accountable for the wellbeing of their children and in turn requires children to take care of their parents in their old age (Barnett and Whiteside 2006: 210). Without this familial welfare system, society and the state are left to bear the burden.[9] In the absence of effective national health care the brunt of this burden of care most often falls to the women in affected communities.

The gender implications of HIV and AIDS go well beyond that. In impoverished circumstances, women's disadvantaged positions mean that they often experience the epidemic with greater intensity. With limited rights and means of support women may resort to bartering or selling sex to ensure their wellbeing. Women are also biologically more at risk, being twice as likely to acquire HIV during intercourse than heterosexual men (UNAIDS 2009). In many communities women are also perceived to be the carriers of disease as they are the first to notice their illness when they fall pregnant and visit clinics (Marais 2005: 15). Moreover, in the case of pregnancy, women are the ones who are required to deal with the added burden and responsibility of protecting their unborn child from becoming infected.

AIDS has also made itself deeply felt in South Africa's economy. These effects can be assessed on two levels: first there are the direct costs associated with ill-health and premature death like spending on health care, funerals and the costs incurred as a result of increased sick leave and diminished overall productivity. Secondly, the consequences resulting from a changed demographic structure like a smaller working class, more dependents and fewer consumers need to be considered (De Waal 2003: 6). In a preliminary report, Arndt and Lewis (2000)

9 UNAIDS (2006) estimated the total amount of AIDS orphans in 2006 at over 1.2 million. See Stein (2003) for a review of the impacts of HIV and AIDS on children and orphans.

have suggested that by 2015 the South African economy would have lost 17 per cent of its productivity due to AIDS.

AIDS also dramatically alters the political landscape. A study by Strand et al. (2004) warns that AIDS could 'undermine South Africa's democratic project'. The reduced national life expectancy affects governance on two levels: it decreases the number of voters and it threatens to diminish the institutional capacity of a state by killing off experienced and well-networked staff (De Waal 2003: 11, 15). Institutional capacity is further eroded as the South African epidemic is claiming a large number of public educators and civil workers (Peltzer 2008: 103–4).

Accusations of inaction and denial

The South African AIDS epidemic is formidable both in terms of its extent as well as its effects. But this need not have been the case, critics argue, as the means of addressing the epidemic and buffering its potentially devastating effects abound. Many of these have been available to government since the onset of the epidemic. These responses may range from prevention programmes, AIDS awareness and education campaigns to counselling and medical support for the sick.

The development of anti-retroviral drugs (ARVs) in the mid-1990s has made even more effective options available for responding to the epidemic. ARVs have practically rendered AIDS a medically manageable chronic condition (Cameron 2000: 10). However, whilst some countries embraced this opportunity and began ARV rollout as soon as the drugs were made available, in South Africa government has been strongly opposed to ARV rollout. The reasons that successive South African governments have given for their reluctance have ranged from rational, financial arguments to more controversial suspicions over the science of AIDS, arguing for instance that ARVs are toxic or that HIV does not cause AIDS. The latter arguments speak directly to the tenets of AIDS dissidence or denialism.[10] It eventually took a Constitutional Court ruling to force the South African government to issue Nevirapine for mother-to-child treatment prevention (MTCTP) in 2003. Highly Active Antiretroviral Therapy (HAART) was only made available the following year (Nattrass 2004: 41).

Until late 2008, in spite of over a thousand South Africans dying of AIDS every day, rollout continued to be hopelessly lethargic. By December 2007, according to the WHO (2008: 120), only 28 per cent of the population in need of ARVs were receiving it. This compares dismally with rollout levels of 79 per cent in Botswana and 88 per cent in Namibia. Furthermore, in South Africa only an estimated 57 per cent of women needing MTCTP were covered, compared with 96 per cent in Botswana and 64 per cent in Namibia. It is generally agreed that treatment rollout should never have been delayed in this manner. As Kalichman (2009: 127)

10 Refer to Chapter 3 for a clarification of the difference between denial and denialism.

recently remarked, 'denialism has plagued South Africa nearly as badly as the epidemic itself'.

Critics have responded to this treatment lethargy with outrage. Nattrass (2004: 41) for instance has called this a 'sorry tale of missed opportunities, inadequate analysis, bureaucratic failure and political mismanagement'. The UN Special Envoy for HIV and AIDS in Africa, Stephen Lewis (2006: 3) has noted more strongly that:

> [South Africa] is the only country in Africa...whose government is still obtuse, dilatory and negligent about rolling out treatment. It is the only country in Africa whose government continues to propound theories more worthy of a lunatic fringe than of a concerned and compassionate state...The government has a lot to atone for.

In a recent study from Harvard University, Chigwedere et al. (2008) accuse the South African government of acting as 'a major obstacle' in providing medication to people with HIV and AIDS. They used modelling to calculate the lives that were lost through government's failure to initiate a 'feasible and timely' ARV treatment programme. According to their calculations, in the period between 2000 and 2005 at least 330,000 lives could have been saved had the government reacted appropriately. These statistics have led to repeated calls for an AIDS-specific Truth and Reconciliation Commission (TRC) that would investigate these unnecessary deaths and hold the government accountable.[11]

The purpose of this book

Clearly, Thabo Mbeki's controversial views on AIDS and his governments' objections to treatment rollout have caused great outcry. It is not surprising then that it has become common practice to allocate most of the blame for South Africa's AIDS epidemic to Mbeki and his governments' denialist stance. This appears to have reached its zenith only very recently with public calls for Mbeki to be tried for genocide.

This book challenges the commonly held perception that it is for the most part 'Mbeki's fault' and argues instead, that matters of blame and denial are not that easily resolved. This is particularly true of events that stretch across extended periods of time – known as 'long-wave events'. As an alternative to simply blaming Mbeki, the authors propose an investigation into government inaction that extends beyond the more recent incidents of denialism and inadequate treatment rollout, associated with Mbeki. Government inaction prior to Mbeki may not seem as blatant as the more recent treatment lethargy associated with Mbeki's governments, but prevention options were still at hand that, if implemented effectively, could

11 See Karim (2009) as well as *The Lancet* (2006).

have helped curb the surge in infection and death that unfolded during Mbeki's two terms in office. With a more historical take on the South African epidemic, the authors hope to shed new light on the dynamics of blame and denial that are implicated in the South African epidemic.

A cursory review of government action suggests that long before ARVs were readily and cheaply available and prior to Mbeki's controversial handling of the epidemic, South African officials failed to adequately respond to the epidemic. A nearly exponential growth of HIV infections since 1982 testifies to a history of ineffective action and reaction that significantly predates the Mbeki governments' grappling with AIDS science. Whilst ARVs are vital in treating and managing existing infections, effectively stemming the epidemic requires a significant effort at preventing new infections from occurring in the first place. This prevention option was available to the South African government long before the development of effective and affordable treatment in the late 1990s. And yet the official response in the years just after the first two cases were recorded seemed to be based almost exclusively on rhetoric and propaganda as the apartheid government assured the white public that they were not at risk since HIV was limited to homosexual white men, commercial sex workers and intravenous drug users. Even when it became quite clear that the epidemic had made a heterosexual transition, putting the vast majority of the population at risk, the government, instead of retaliating with prevention efforts, government response continued to be mostly rhetorical. Instead, this time they singled out the general black population as primary carriers of HIV (Grundlingh 2001: 125–6; Van der Vliet 2001: 156).

Towards the end of the 1980s South African officials increasingly acknowledged the epidemic, now publically announcing plans to counter it. But their promises continued to translate into very little action. At the time the political concerns of the day overshadowed what appeared to be a relatively minor concern by comparison (Grundlingh 2001: 128). When the transition to democracy ushered in a new era of policy making and open discussion, government put pen to paper. The National AIDS Convention of South Africa (NACOSA) was founded in 1992 and went on to draft South Africa's first National AIDS Plan (NAP) in 1994. Although it was commended as an impeccable document, the NAP overestimated the 'new' South Africa's institutional capacity and subsequently failed to make significant inroads in the fight against AIDS (see Chapters 4 and 5). HIV and AIDS again appeared to have fallen by the wayside. By 1997 Mandela had been in office for three years when he finally made his first major statement on AIDS (Nattrass 2007: 40).

Noting government's continued failure to effectively curb the spread of HIV and stem the epidemic, a number of critics have pointed to a history of lethargy and possibly even denial. Heywood (2004: 2), has remarked that the transition to democracy and ensuing social reconstruction have at times been 'accompanied by attempts to ignore, hide and marginalise the advance of the HIV and AIDS epidemic'. Looking further back, Furlong and Ball (2005: 128) have argued that the same 'gap between rhetoric and reality, lack of political will, funding and generally slow policy development and implementation' that characterised the post-1994 governments' responses were also present in government response before that. These arguments point to a history of inadequate official response that goes back to the initial years of the epidemic. This continued failure to address the epidemic effectively has given rise to further speculations that successive South African governments might have been in a 'state of denial' about the epidemic (Van Niekerk 2001: 149).

Whilst accusations of government denial may have often be expressed in discussions of South Africa's handling of the AIDS epidemic (in particular with reference to its more recent actions), not much investigation has thus far been done into the dynamics of blame and denial in the epidemic. Moreover, when cast against South Africa's turbulent political history and in light of the initial lack of scientific knowledge about AIDS, theories of early government denial may be questionable.

Taking the unique characteristics of the epidemic into account, this book undertakes to investigate whether there have indeed been distinct and serious instances of South African government AIDS denial and if so, whether these instances have been frequent enough to warrant suggestions that the government has been in a state of denial over the epidemic since its onset in 1982. Most discussions of the South African government's denial in the epidemic have thus far been focused on the disavowal of mainstream AIDS science, or AIDS denialism. Denial as a reaction to the epidemic can, however, go far beyond contesting scientific fact. This book attempts to cast its gaze wider to investigate government denial of AIDS as a whole, including rationalisations and disavowals that extend to cultural, financial and political arguments. In so doing, this analysis goes far beyond merely examining government action for signs of denial. By uncovering some of the political pressures exerted by a long-wave event like HIV and AIDS and considering the uncertainty and devastation posed by the epidemic, this book provides valuable insight into the mechanisms of blame and denial (however subtle) that could have been at play in South Africa since 1982.

The structure of this book

Chapter 2: The South African AIDS Epidemic This is an important contextualising chapter that sets out the epidemiological evolution and the current status of the South African AIDS epidemic. The chapter also contains a discussion of the key drivers/determinants of the local epidemic, as well as its impact.

Chapter 3: Developing a Theory of Government AIDS Denial This chapter formulates a theory of government denial and conceptualises a typology of official denial (as devised by Stanley Cohen) that is applied as an analytical tool throughout the discussion to make sense of AIDS denial in South Africa.

Part I: A History of the Official Response Part I consists of Chapters 4–6, which set out a chronological political history of the South African epidemic. These chapters inform the analysis of AIDS denial in Part II. Throughout this historical narrative, possible instances of government denial are earmarked and then taken up thematically in Part II. Chapters 4–6 are therefore chronological and sequential units of analysis, whereas Part II applies elements/themes of a denial typology as units of analysis.

Chapter 4: Past is Prologue: Apartheid Responses to AIDS This chapter describes the Botha and De Klerk (apartheid) governments' responses by focusing on three phases of response: (1) the 'silent' phase (1982–88), (2) flux and reconceptualisation (1989–92) and (3) the democratisation of the official response to AIDS (1992–94).

Chapter 5: The Mandela Government's Response to AIDS This chapter describes how the idealism of the new government's AIDS response gave way first to pragmatism and then to disillusionment and denial. This led to a comedy of errors regarding AIDS governance during the last few years of the Mandela government.

Chapter 6: The Two Mbeki Governments' Responses to AIDS This chapter consists of two sections. The first section describes the first Mbeki government's (1999–2004) nascent flirtation with and gradual defence of AIDS denialism and the second section explains how this led to the institutionalisation of the denial of AIDS as policy during the intractable second Mbeki administration (2004–08).

Part II: Making Sense of Official AIDS Denial Part II consists of Chapters 7–10, where Cohen's typology official denial that was discussed in Chapter 3 is used as an analytical tool to cast more light on the instances of possible denial that have been identified in the chronological outline of successive South African governments' response to the epidemic. The discussion now takes on a thematic structure to address topics that may have informed government denial. These themes include classic official denial, counter-offensive denial, partial acknowledgement and an overview of the politics of denial as a whole. This section ends with a general conclusion to the book.

Chapter 7: Classic Official Denial This chapter identifies three kinds of official denial and then applies these to the historical evolution set out in Part I.

Chapter 8: Counter-offensive Denial and Partial Acknowledgement This chapter builds on the conceptualisation of official denial by applying counter-offensive denial and partial acknowledgement as two complementary strategies used in the construction of AIDS denial. These are applied to the history of official AIDS responses in South Africa discussed in Part I.

Chapter 9: The Politics of Denial This chapter consolidates the incremental analysis in Part II by clarifying the motives behind the denial of AIDS, as well as by making explicit the dynamics of blame, accountability, victimhood and the construction of 'bogeymen' in the history of AIDS in South Africa.

Chapter 10: Conclusion This chapter summarises the key findings of the book and identifies areas for future research. Importantly, the Conclusion also provides a graphic representation of a denial timeline and superimposes it on top of a chronology of the official history of the South African epidemic.

Chapter 2
The South African AIDS Epidemic

Introduction

Understanding the unique nature of the AIDS epidemic is important for discussing the dynamics of blame and denial in the South African government's response to HIV and AIDS. Knowing the extent and severity of the epidemic further informs the importance of investigating official denial in South Africa's HIV and AIDS story. In this light one could argue that the gravity of government denial is implicitly tied to the severity of the South African AIDS epidemic. In other words, the lesser the threat posed by HIV and AIDS to South African society, economy and politics, the more trivial government denial would be. The opposite also holds true. With this in mind, achieving the most accurate depiction of the epidemic possible is of crucial importance. Only against this outline will the significance of investigating accusations of denial become apparent.

Grasping the full extent of the South African epidemic, however, is a formidable undertaking. Data can be a useful source of information, depicting the scale of the epidemic, illustrating its progress and helping to predict and measure its impacts. However, data may also be misleading, inaccurate or simply hard to come by. Even perfectly accurate data can only paint a limited picture – focusing on certain aspects and leaving out others. Accurately depicting the epidemic is further complicated by the long-wave nature of HIV and AIDS. South Africa has also offered a unique terrain to the HI virus. The socio-political context during apartheid and prevailing social practices have contributed to the rampant spread of HIV and AIDS.

This chapter considers all of these points – the constraints of data, the nature of long-wave events and the unique South African context – before moving on to give an overview of the impact of HIV and AIDS on South Africa's social environment, economy and politics. Once this has been achieved, the discussion can move on to allegations of government denial.

Understanding epidemic curves and long-wave events

Launching head-first into a rigorous discussion of the South African epidemic, replete with harrowing demographic figures and the findings of landmark studies, would add little value to this discussion without the necessary context and knowledge of the AIDS epidemic. At first glance, for instance, the recent UNAIDS *Report on the global AIDS epidemic's* announcement that HIV prevalence in South Africa may have stabilised (although it is at an 'extraordinarily high level') seems like nothing but good news (UNAIDS 2008: 15). However, once viewed against the backdrop of epidemic curves and long-wave events, this becomes a much less optimistic finding. Epidemiology suggests that slowed infection is probably more likely the cause of infection reaching a point of natural saturation, whilst long-wave studies offer the disheartening prospect that the worst of the impact of HIV infections is still to come.

Epidemic curves

A typical epidemic curve is S-shaped (as Figure 2.1 below illustrates). As a virus is introduced to a society, the initial infection rate is slow. However, once it has been allowed to spread, a critical mass of infection is reached and the infection rate increases rapidly as the epidemic reaches its full force. The infection rate again slows down when most of the people that have been exposed to the virus have become infected.

Those left uninfected are either not susceptible to the virus, or simply lucky. The curve then turns downwards, marking the final phase of the epidemic. This decline in new infections is brought about either by people getting better, or more grimly, by an increased incidence of death that leaves behind significantly fewer people that can be infected (Barnett and Whiteside 2006: 52).

This natural progression of epidemics means that the apparent 'levelling off' of the South African epidemic is more likely to be the result of HIV infection having reached a point of natural saturation than the product of successful intervention (Gouws and Abdool Karim 2008: 48).

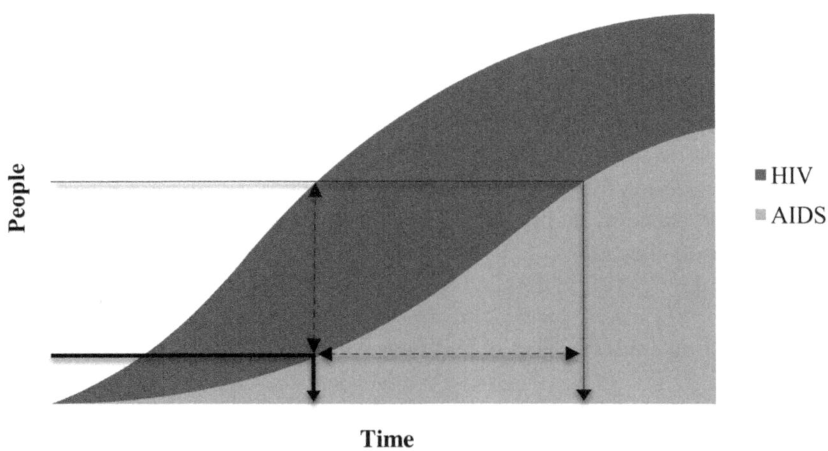

Figure 2.1 HIV and AIDS epidemic curves

Source: Adapted from Whiteside and Sunter (2000: 27).

Long-wave events

Still, this levelling-off does not mean that the worst of the epidemic is over. Unlike fast-spreading viruses that cause death within a few days of infection, the case of HIV and AIDS is different. Because infection and illness can be between five and eight years apart (even up to ten years), properly illustrating the full effect of HIV and AIDS requires two epidemic curves (as indicated in Figure 2.1). The first S-curve signifies HIV infection. The second curve represents the onset of AIDS. It is identical in shape to the first curve, but, in keeping with the delayed onset of full-blown AIDS, lags between five and eight years behind the first (Whiteside and Sunter 2000: 26–7).

In terms of effect, HIV infections are unremarkable as the infected person's system is not yet significantly weakened. Whilst the impact of the HIV curve goes largely unnoticed, quite the opposite holds true for the AIDS curve. This is because shortly after patients are diagnosed with AIDS, without treatment, they fall gravely ill and die. In this regard the second curve presents the point at which the real impact of the epidemic manifests. Therefore, when statistics report a slowed infection rate, they are actually referring to the first, HIV curve. That same slow-down in infection will thus only really be observed in five to eight years, by which time the infections would have developed into AIDS illness (illustrated by the dotted lines in Figure 2.1).

This delayed effect means that AIDS belongs to a special category of occurrences known as 'long-wave events'. HIV and AIDS is not a disaster that strikes overnight like a tsunami or cholera (or the H1N1 swine flu virus in April 2009). Unlike these short-wave emergencies that play out over a few hours or days and therefore are much more tangible, long-wave events like HIV and AIDS run their course much more insidiously over many years (Barnett 2006: 302). Whilst short-term disasters have immediate consequences that require immediate responses and attract a great deal of international attention and support, long-term events pass so slowly that they are often integrated into people's lives as they learn to 'cope' with its effects. Often these long-wave events do not get noticed much beyond that.

Because of their gradual, creeping nature, long-wave events require a response that is very different from the normal short-term emergency reaction. As a result, governments often find themselves ill prepared and bewildered by the prospect of such a long-lasting event. This has certainly been the case with the AIDS epidemic. The study of long-wave events can lend a great deal of insight into the reactions of governments to the epidemic as well as offer some important insight into the nature of the AIDS epidemic itself. Barnett (2006: 302–3) gives the following description of long-wave events:

- Their starting points are usually unknown.
- Once there is awareness of the event, its dynamic and effects, the event is usually already well on its way. This means that intervention may take a long time to yield results – if the event can be stopped at all.

- Addressing the implications and long-term ramifications of long-wave events requires long-term thinking. This is very different from the type of thinking leaders and civil society are used to as they typically deal almost exclusively with short-wave events.
- It is extremely difficult to get people in positions of power to recognise these events, to mobilise adequate resources to deal with them and to take appropriate action. This comes as these events fall outside the normal time horizons of politicians and business strategists, for whom 'long-term' usually means five years. Long-wave events, on the other hand, are likely to cover many decades and probably periods much longer than that. This is one of the main reasons why these events are difficult to halt.
- Managing the consequences of long-wave events makes novel demands on leaders and society. Moreover, existing experience cannot always be drawn on to suggest how to respond to these events.
- Consequently, dealing with them lies beyond most political and administrative capacities; and
- When these events are 'discovered' they are thought of and reacted to as 'emergencies'. This gives way to the possibility that hasty, rash actions taken for good in the short term might make the situation worse in the long term.

Together, knowledge of epidemic curves and long-wave events add important depth to fully understanding the extent and effects of the South African epidemic. This also allows for a more accurate description of the real gravity of the situation. Statistics suggest that around 5.7 million South Africans are HIV-positive. With an estimated overall population of around 48.7 million, this means that over 10 per cent of South Africans are HIV-positive (Statistics SA 2008: 3). These infections are still latent, in the sense that they are yet to turn into actual illness. The strain that nearly 6 million ill people will have on the country's health infrastructure, economy and politics in a few years' time is bound to be immense and at this point, practically unfathomable. All of the ensuing discussions on impact can only attempt to predict these effects in a future of uncertainty. Moreover, as the study of long-wave events demonstrates, governments are not designed to deal with crises of this duration. Budgets cannot be allocated for health care in eight years' time. Action must be taken now, but with the consequence of inaction looming too far ahead in the future to instil the necessary sense of urgency, incentives are slight.

Demography and statistics

The South African AIDS epidemic is the best studied and documented one in Africa. Still the estimates and accounts differ, sometimes vastly (Marais 2005: 27). During the epidemic's first ten years, the statistics for AIDS in South

Africa were unreliable. Official statistics seemed to severely understate the epidemic. In 1992 official records reported 26 AIDS deaths nationally, whilst one hospital in Kwa-Zulu Natal alone recorded 153 AIDS deaths (and this only in the first nine months of that year) (Furlong and Ball 2005: 133). Also, a lack of reliable data sometimes leaves researchers no choice but to use data of inferior quality (Whiteside et al. 2005: 33). Projections and estimates are also sometimes presented and interpreted with an unwarranted degree of certainty (Marais 2005: 27).

AIDS data presents itself in various forms, each with its own advantages and shortcomings. In order to get as much of the whole picture of HIV and AIDS in South Africa as possible, it is important to understand what each of these types of data brings to the table.

AIDS has significant impacts for populations. Demography, the study of populations and their dynamics, therefore offers some important insight into the extent of the epidemic. However, demography is often not accurate enough to paint a full picture of impact and effect. Barnett and Whiteside (2006: 180) point to three problems resulting from demographic data. The first takes issue with the difference between an event and a process. Whilst HIV and AIDS is a process concerning the deterioration of health and eventual death, with a great deal of resulting consequences, demographers can only quantify events – like deaths or orphaning. This means that only crude numbers are recorded whilst other salient issues like the selling off of household assets in the event of an illness, lost hours of productivity or decreased school attendance go unnoticed. Secondly, demographic surveys have a very wide focus – investigating provinces, municipal districts or entire nations at a time, whilst AIDS is often very concentrated, clustered in households or villages and therefore felt more severely by certain communities than a nation-wide census might reflect. Finally, the frequency at which these data are obtained is often too far apart, rendering much of the information outdated and of very little value.

Similarly, other kinds of statistics can also fall short of the standards of accurate and reliable information. As Whiteside et al. (2005: 21) suggest, surveys can be wrong and/or miscalculated. Data could be subjected to political motive and be obscured or withheld by governments (Whiteside et al. 2005: 22). Many HIV and AIDS illnesses are also simply not recorded as either the ill do not come into contact with official medical services or the stigmatisation around the issue persuades the medical staff to report the case as something other than HIV and AIDS (Whiteside et al. 2005: 23).

Still, data allows for an opportunity to both understand and convey to others the sheer scale of the epidemic. By way of example, Figure 1.2 draws on data collected in an actuarial study conducted in 2006 by Dorrington et al. (2006) and allows for an illustration of the immense growth of the epidemic in the last 15 years. Combining these figures with knowledge of epidemic curves and long-wave events can assist in illustrating in which phase of the epidemic South Africa is at present. The *Total HIV+* curve represents the first S-curve of the epidemic, whilst the curve indicating *Cumulative AIDS deaths* represents the second. In keeping with the typical epidemic model, the *Cumulative AIDS deaths* curve can be expected to rise until it has reached the level of the *Total HIV+* curve, or put differently, until all HIV-positive individuals have fallen ill and died.

What makes these impending mortalities even more devastating is the fact that AIDS hits those individuals the hardest who are of a productive and working age. Statistics can help generate a better understanding. According to the Dorrington et al. (2006) study, prevalence amongst South African men aged 30 to 34 was as high as 26.5 per cent and reached a maximum of 32.5 per cent amongst women aged 25 to 29. It is here that the crux of the impact of the AIDS epidemic can be found – it increases morbidity and mortality in populations precisely where they are typically low – namely in the middle ages (Barnett and Whiteside 2006: 172). This means that, if left untreated, at least a quarter of the backbone of South African society – the income generators, those who care for children and the elderly, educators, civil servants – will fall ill and die prematurely.

Again the impact of AIDS is shown most effectively with the help of data. Figures 2.2 and 2.3 (below) are based on information contained in a Statistics South Africa report by Anderson and Phillips (2006: 10) and show increases in male and female mortality respectively. The report found that increases in mortality between 1997 and 2004 were concentrated in the younger ages, specifically 20–44 years and especially for females. Furthermore, between 1997 and 2004 the death rate for females aged 25–34 increased more than four-fold (from 941 deaths per 100,000 to 4,252 deaths per 100,000). For men in the same age group the death rate more than doubled (from 1,442 deaths per 100,000 to 3,199 per 100,000).

This increase in mortality has led to a decline in population growth from a high of 2.7 per cent in 1992 to an estimated 0.7 per cent in 2008 (Dorrington et al. 2006: 21). Although not all of these mortalities can be attributed to HIV and AIDS,

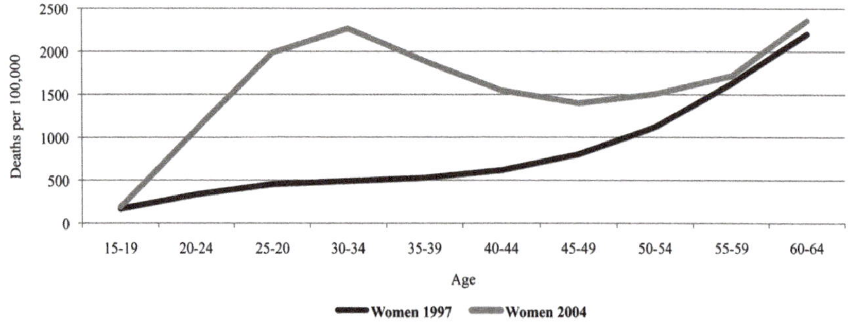

Figure 2.2 Increase in male mortality

Source: Anderson and Philips (2006).

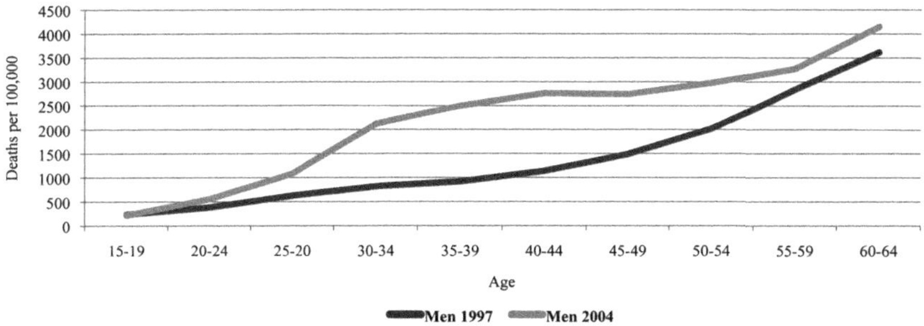

Figure 2.3 Increase in female mortality
Source: Anderson and Philips (2006).

since 1982 AIDS is estimated to have claimed the lives of over 2,535,836 South Africans (Dorrington et al. 2006: 21). Since 2006 roughly 900 South Africans have died of AIDS daily, so in 2010 this total cumulative number of South African AIDS dead is probably well in excess of three million.

AIDS changes the *structure* of populations. Whilst the Black Death, for instance, was indiscriminate and therefore killed people uniformly and randomly, AIDS is concentrated amongst the most productive members of society (Barnett and Clement 2005: 237). Natural disasters and wars also kill indiscriminately whilst famines tend to kill the very young, the very old and the frail and sickly (Marais 2005: 10). The people killed by AIDS are not only the breadwinners of the country but also the majority of voters as well as the caregivers of the young and the old. This has serious social, political and economic implications.

Whilst we suggest above that data are not always to be taken at face value, data can significantly increase understanding of the scale and potential impact of the epidemic (as the figures above have). Even so, it is important to remain mindful of the fact that data do not always portray the absolute truth and may be misleading. As the next section will show, inaccurate data made the epidemic appear much less harmful in the initial years. However, irrespective of statistical inaccuracy, insufficient or inaccurate data should never be an excuse for policy makers and officials to contest the seriousness of the epidemic (Furlong and Ball 2005: 133).

Statistics and the evolution of the South African AIDS epidemic

Whilst the statistics cited above paint the picture of a lethal virus that will decimate[1] the population and potentially compromise development and political

1 To say that the South African population is being decimated is an understatement. The term 'decimate' is intended to refer to the loss of one in ten people (although, over time it has been applied in more general terms to suggest an overall sense of destruction). If, as Statistics

Table 2.1 Reported South African AIDS cases

1982	1983	1984	1985	1986	1987	1988	1989	1990	1991	1992
2	4	8	8	34	51	98	184	345	549	887

Source: UNAIDS (2004: 6).

stability (that is, without adequate intervention), the South African AIDS epidemic has had a slow and silent start. In fact, throughout the 1980s it seemed to pose no considerable threat, confined for the most part to marginal groups like men who have sex with men (MSM), sex workers and mine workers. However, as unremarkable statistics bred complacency, the makings for a perfect epidemic were already in place. These included the migrant worker system as well as the inadequate access to health care afforded to the black majority by the apartheid government (Heywood 2008: 373).

The first two recorded South African AIDS deaths were reported in 1982. As the UNAIDS statistics in Table 2.1 indicate, over the course of the next decade the number of reported AIDS cases grew exponentially. But still the numbers were low, creating the false impression that there was no real problem.

But whilst these statistics suggested the problem was still under control, HIV was spreading rampantly, far away from the watchful eye of clinicians and statisticians. According to Dorrington et al. (2006: 21), in 1992, ten years after the first two AIDS deaths were reported, 159,726 South Africans were HIV-positive, 1,726 were ill with AIDS and the epidemic had already claimed 2,128 lives. The official statistics as reported by UNAIDS suggest an entirely different picture.

To make matters worse, as the incidence of AIDS illness in clinics and hospitals began to increase noticeably, HIV infections continued to spread under the radar. As these infections would only manifest in full-blown illness in a few years to come, they went largely unnoticed at the time, creating the false impression that the epidemic was still under control and therefore also appearing to eliminate the need for a large-scale response. In the meantime, spreading infections formed 'a wave of future suffering, cost and death' that would come crashing down quite unexpectedly in the future (Whiteside and Barnett 2006: 20). This is a typical characteristic of long-wave events.[2] As Marais (2005: 26) points out, it is only once people fall ill and die that the impact becomes more visible. This phase only really began in South Africa in the late 1990s.

South Africa suggest, 5.7 million people out of a total population of 48.7 million are HIV-positive, then nearly 12 per cent or one in eight South Africans could face death if there is no intervention (Statistics SA 2003: 3). This is beyond the scale of technical decimation.

2 Earlier in the chapter Barnett (2006: 302) points out that once people become aware of the presence of long-wave events, their effects and dynamic, it takes a long time to stop it or slow it down, if this is still even possible.

The fact that in its early years the epidemic was severely underreported and understated has been a significant contributing factor to its unchecked spread. It was only once the African National Congress (ANC) came to power that AIDS became a serious talking point on the agenda and by that time much of the damage had already been done (Grundlingh 2001: 144–53). However, government negligence in the face of insufficient and inaccurate data cannot alone account for the enormous extent of the epidemic. When the HI virus arrived in South Africa the country presented a unique and ideal breeding ground. Amongst others, the political climate of the day bred exclusion of the black majority, vulnerable groups were stigmatised and the migrant labour system led to the creation of vast and uncontrolled sexual networks. Moreover, a number of prevailing social and political issues have ensured that the virus continues to spread rapidly even after the termination of the apartheid system.

Why is the South African epidemic so severe?

Imagine going to a South African cinema to see a movie. There are 15 rows in the cinema. Each row has 16 seats and the theatre is filled to capacity. If this were a family film in which the audience is made up of men and women of all ages, then statistically one in eight people in the cinema would be HIV-positive – enough to fill almost the first two rows. If it were a drama that appealed to a more mature audience between the ages of 20 and 64, then statistically nearly one in five people would be HIV-positive – enough, this time, to fill three rows. If, on the other hand, it were an action film and the audience was mostly made up of men aged between 30 and 40, then statistically one in four would be HIV-positive; they would be taking up nearly four rows. Or, if it were a romantic comedy that women aged between 25 and 35 were watching, then statistically, nearly one in three people would be HIV-positive – that is either the person to your left, or to your right, or you![3]

The same scenario would play out very differently in, for instance, Brazil with an audience aged between 14 and 50. In this case the HIV-positive people would not be able to fill a row (around 14 people). In the UK amongst the same audience demographic the total number of HIV-positive people would be less than five![4] These figures stand out in stark comparison to South Africa. The latter has the largest number of HIV infections in the world (UNAIDS 2007: 16) accounting for 10 per cent of the global burden of infection (Gouws and Abdool Karim 2008: 55).

It is generally agreed that government inaction alone cannot be held accountable for the sheer scale of the South African epidemic. When HIV

3 This illustration makes use of figures provided by Dorrington et al. (2006). The theatre size is based on the average South African cinema in which there are 15 rows with 16 seats in each row.

4 Figures are based on UNAIDS 2008 prevalence rates.

arrived in South Africa, society presented an almost ideal breeding ground for the virus. Many of these factors continue to make South African society uniquely vulnerable to infection.

Apartheid's legacy of poverty and migratory labour

Poverty in many ways is (or at least, should be) the point of departure for any discussion about HIV and AIDS in South Africa. A general environment of endemic poverty gives rise to most other factors that lead to the rapid and unchecked spread of disease. Limited or no public services like running water, sanitation and waste management as well as limited access to health care mean that diseases spread rampantly and for the most part unchecked. Poor nutrition weakens people's immune systems, making them more susceptible to opportunistic illness and extending the time it takes for them to get well again. Poverty can also give rise to increased incidences of criminality, including rape and drug abuse. Poverty also fosters economic inequalities between men and women, often leaving women disempowered and vulnerable to positions in which they have little choice but to resort to sex in exchange for basic goods. These are only some of the ways in which poverty can aggravate the spread of HIV.[5]

As Marais (2005: 101) points out, 'AIDS does not afflict all…in equal measure; it feeds off and aggravates existing inequalities'. In South Africa these inequalities are severe. The legacy of apartheid means that poverty is a racialised and politicised issue. As part of South Africa's policy of 'separate development' the black population was politically and materially marginalised. Black South Africans received only a fraction of the health services and educational opportunities that were afforded to the white minority. This begot a general ignorance towards issues of STIs as well as an overall low level of literacy. The confinement of the black population to homelands where adequate housing was insufficient further encouraged the unchecked spread of HIV and ensured that black South Africans would continue to live in impoverished conditions (Grundlingh 2001: 146).

Apart from contributing to the rampant spread of HIV, this legacy of poverty severely hampered initial attempts at raising awareness of HIV and AIDS. Firstly, the high rates of illiteracy meant that any campaigns conducted by means of the written word were redundant. Secondly, because apartheid instilled an innate and understandable suspicion of the state in black South Africans, government efforts at AIDS education were viewed as a means of curbing population growth (Grundlingh 2001: 146). Even after South African democratisation, AIDS remains a hotly contested, highly personal and deeply humiliating subject, particularly for black South Africans.

Through the forced confinement of black South Africans to homelands that were far removed from industry the apartheid government gave the black

5 Also see Kalichman et al. (2006), Halperin and Allen (2001), Whiteside (2004) and Van Niekerk (2001).

population little choice but to migrate to urban areas (and mines) where they would find employment. Once in the cities the workers had little choice but to spend months on end away from their wives and girlfriends, living in single-sex hostels known as compounds. Sources of amusement and channels for escapism were limited to alcohol and prostitutes. Coupled with the worker's limited knowledge of STDs (thanks to their restricted education) this system created an ideal breeding ground for HIV. When the migrant workers returned home to their families, they too would be exposed to the virus. Soon migrant workers found themselves both victims and vectors in a sexual network that rapidly spread HIV across the country (Jochelson, Mothibeli and Ledger 1992; Lurie 2000).

Biomedical factors

HIV is known as a free-riding infection that targets weakened immune systems. This ties in closely with issues of poverty and in the South African case, poverty in turn relates to issues of race. Because of inadequate healthcare and poor living standards, it is estimated that around half of the black population in South Africa has at some point had TB. This leaves their immune systems scarred for life and more vulnerable to HIV infection. Poor healthcare and desperate conditions also contribute to the rampant spread of STDs (further compounded by the migrant labour system). Sexually transmitted infections (STIs), in particular those causing genital ulcering, significantly increase the chances of acquiring HIV, as well as of transmitting it (Corey et al. 2004). Research has also shown that the predominant subtype of the HI virus in South Africa, HIV-1 Clade C, is the most likely to develop drug-resistant mutations (Calms 2008).

Furthermore, most South African men are not circumcised. There is compelling evidence that circumcised men are much less likely to contract the HI virus than their uncircumcised counterparts.[6] However, whilst circumcision can decrease a man's chance of contracting the HI virus by up to 60 per cent, sexual behaviour still has a lot to account for.

Issues of gender, relationships and culture

Given the intimate manner in which HIV is spread it is not surprising that HIV and AIDS are tied closely to issues of gender and relationships. These issues in turn are informed by the broader cultural and social context. In South Africa poverty has been a significant force in shaping this context, as well as to a lesser extent the apartheid system along with existing traditional beliefs.

---

6 A number of studies have been conducted on circumcision. See for instance Halperin and Epstein (2007), Lagarde et al. (2003) and Weiss, Quigley and Hayes (2000). Whilst there is evidence that male circumcision provides some measure of protection for men, it is doubtful whether male circumcision has any effect on reducing the chances of HIV transmission to women (see Baeten, Celum and Coates (2009) as well as Wawer et al. (2009)).

Under apartheid women were afforded minimal rights. These were even more limited for black women who were not only economically powerless but also had virtually no rights and were considered the legal minors of their husbands. Relinquishing rights to this extent is often coupled with a sense of sexual disempowerment in which women are expected to submit themselves to the expectations of their 'benefactors'. These women are therefore seldom in a position in which they can insist on condom use. This kind of gender inequality, although considerably less severe than under apartheid, persists to this day.

That said, Leclerc-Madlala (2003) cautions that women's recent resorting to transactional sex is not always a matter of necessity and survival. In Leclerc-Madlala's studies women have admitted to resorting to transactional sex as a means of achieving material gains that are not considered a necessity (acquiring, for instance, mobile phones or jewellery). Sex in this case becomes a matter of satisfying wants more than needs. The men that these women seek out to be their benefactors are often considerably older. In the case of such intergenerational sex women tend to be less likely to insist on condom use and therefore face a higher risk of becoming infected (Leclerc-Madlala 2008).

Studies have also revealed that African men and women tend to have multiple concurrent sexual partnerships – in other words more than one long-term relationship at a time (this involves both casual concurrent partnerships and more formal polygamous arrangements). As trust is established over time these relationships often entail practicing unprotected sex. Both partners are therefore at a high risk of contracting the virus as either is part of an extended and active sexual network (Halperin and Epstein 2007). This is not to suggest that black South Africans are more promiscuous than white people anywhere else; sexual practices differ. In most Western cultures people tend have multiple short-term relationships or so-called one-night-stands. In long-term relationships, partners establish mutual trust and often waive condom use, whilst during one-night-stands partners are more likely to insist on condom use.

Poverty also fosters situations where crime and violence are rife. Often this violence is of a sexual nature. South Africa has a shockingly high incidence of rape.[7] Some have suggested that sexual violence is a product of poverty which creates a crisis of male identity. Rape then becomes men's only escape from powerlessness – the only space in which they able to express their dominance and exercise superiority. Whilst the underlying motivators for sexual violence in themselves could be the subject of a book, it suffices to say here that as a whole this culture of rape contributes significantly to the spread of HIV. Rape leads to genital injury, increasing the probability of infection. Also, sexual assault is often committed by more than one offender. In the case of such gang rape, risk of exposure increases significantly. It has also been suggested that sexual assault may lead to riskier sexual behaviour in the survivor of the rape/assault (Marks 2008: 48–9).

---

7 Rape has been described as endemic to South Africa (BBC 2002). A recent study suggests that one in four South African men have committed rape (Jewkes et al. 2009).

A number of cultural practices and myths further entrench vulnerability to HIV. For instance, a frightening number of South Africans believe that having sex with a virgin can cure AIDS. The practice of polygamy or of rites related to death (like a widower marrying his deceased wife's sister) also increase exposure to HIV – especially if the spouse died of AIDS (Shisana 2008: 18).

The impact of the South African AIDS epidemic

Having illustrated some of the unique characteristics of the South African HIV and AIDS epidemic, the role and pitfalls of statistics in portraying its extent, as well as some of the factors that dramatically exacerbate the South African epidemic, we can now more accurately sketch the impacts that HIV and AIDS have (and might have) for South Africa.

Research on the impact of HIV and AIDS is thinner than might be expected. Although impact has become the subject of a growing number of works much of it is still based on speculation with little to no concrete evidence (Mattes and Manning 2004: 191). Whilst much progress has been made in researching treatments and advancing biomedical knowledge of AIDS, social research has in many ways failed to show the same level of advancement. Moreover, even though AIDS is frequently linked to issues of development, the recent critical knowledge gained in development theory and practice is not always being incorporated adequately into AIDS research (Marais 2005: 20). Impact research is also seldom truly multidisciplinary, which hampers achieving a holistic grasp of the true extent on the impact of the epidemic.

That said, a plausible explanation for these shortcomings is at hand. Impact is inherently hard to measure. There are a number of reasons for this. According to Barnett and Whiteside (2006: 713) impact of HIV and AIDS can vary according to level, degree and time. On social and personal levels, like the individual and household levels, impact is severe and early. However, impact on institutions and certain sectors of the economy tends to be less immediate and could vary in severity (Barnett and Whiteside 2006: 173). Consequently, evidence of the impact of HIV and AIDS is largely restricted to those effects that are relatively immediate and severe. Again it is the long-wave nature of AIDS that makes a full understanding of the issue problematic. Whilst for shorter-term impacts like those on the individual there is concrete evidence, for longer-term impacts assessments rely largely on modelling, projections and future scenarios. It is over the long-term, for instance, that AIDS poses a threat to human security; the implications are uncertain (Schneider and Moodie 2002: 4).

Moreover, assessments of HIV and AIDS impact are often hitched to a 'without AIDS' scenario upon which comparison would highlight the extent and severity of the impact. However, as Marais (2005: 35) points out, the 'without AIDS' situation is in effect a counterfactual – it is based on projections and estimates that can never be proven either way. Comparing a world with AIDS to one without it is valuable only in as far as it drives home the severity of the issue. It will, however, never be known whether the 'AIDS free world' looks the way it is made out to be in these hypothetical projections.

The following discussion on impact is structured into three broad categories – social, economic and political impact. Although they are discussed separately, they are all closely related and cumulatively represent the challenge that HIV and AIDS pose to South Africa's development.

Social impacts

The first effects of AIDS are felt at the societal level (Barnett and Whiteside 2006: 197). The most intimate, immediate and strongly felt of these is on the personal level – by those who are HIV-positive. Yet these individual experiences can differ vastly, largely as a result of the resources that persons living with AIDS (PWAs) have at their disposal (Barnett and Whiteside 2006: 198). By way of example, a financially secure individual might, with the help of medication, be able to manage HIV and AIDS to the extent that its effects on his/her lifestyle are minimal – similar to diabetes for most diabetics in the Western world. Conversely, someone less fortunate who cannot afford expensive treatment and care might fall ill with AIDS only a few years after being infected and die less than a year after that. It follows that on the individual level, poverty is a major determining factor of impact.

Family structures That said, individuals do not suffer the effects of HIV and AIDS in isolation. People exist in networks. Consequently their illness and death has serious repercussions for the people within these networks – their immediate families and friends as well as their wider community (Barolsky 2003: 14).

The effects of HIV and AIDS on households or families can be devastating. The intimate nature of HIV and AIDS makes the family unit particularly vulnerable. As they lose members or take on destitute children or sick adults, family structures are forced into a state of constant flux. This could cause the eventual dissolution of the family unit, which in turn can have serious consequences for individuals and society as a whole (Fröhlich 2008: 352). Illness and death also often lead to a drastic reorganisation of relationships and contestation of positions of power within families (Barolsky 2003: 15).

Studying the effect of HIV and AIDS on families and societies can be challenging. For one, the impact on households varies dramatically according to the number of HIV and AIDS cases in a household; the age, gender and income of the ill or deceased person; the original composition of the household and its assets; the attitudes of the community towards helping the needy as well as their access to resources; and finally the broader resources made available by the state and/or NGOs (Barnett and Whiteside 2006: 200).

Instances of AIDS are also often clustered in households, where both parents and some of their offspring could all be infected (Barnett and Whiteside 2006: 198). When the death of one or two parents brings about the dissolution of a household, this data is seldom recorded in household surveys (Barnett and Whiteside 2006: 200). Similarly, communities' ways of coping with the loss of family members (rearranging and reorganising themselves to deal with the dependents that are left behind) also often go unnoticed and unrecorded in surveys. The subtle power shifts and changes that accompany these changes are even more difficult to quantify (Marais 2005: 22).

Implicit assumptions guiding research can also be misleading and distort outcomes. For instance, not all societies are comprised of nuclear family units. For many communities an extended family is the norm, irrespective of instabilities like AIDS (Marais 2005: 22).

What is certain is that HIV and AIDS are dramatically changing the way in which households and families function. As a result a number of new (or unconventional) households are being established. These include households headed by grandparents, enlarged families that take on unrelated orphans, child-headed households, single-parent households, clustered foster care, children in subservient and exploited fostering relationships, displaced or homeless children or gangs (Barnett and Whiteside 2006: 203; also see Fröhlich 2008).

Particularly single (grand)parent households are becoming common. Often these households are of a 'skipped generation' nature in which a single grandparent takes care of orphaned or abandoned children. Although this is not uncommon in situations where either one or both parents migrate to cities to find work, there has been a significant increase in such single parent households. Moreover, as there are no longer two parents to provide financial support for the children, a grandparent or surviving parent is often left to carry the burden of caretaking without additional financial support (Fröhlich 2008: 352–3).

Communities The increased burdens on families invariably spill over into the community as a whole. Again the intensity of the impact of HIV and AIDS on this level is not certain. It is immensely challenging, for instance, to define what constitutes a 'community'. However, in spite of these difficulties, there has been a growing emphasis on the importance of communities in managing the epidemic. The option of home- and community-based care for instance is often considered a cost-effective and more humane means of supporting PWAs than institutionalising or hospitalising them. However, this leads to an increased demand made on already scarce resources in poor communities (Marais 2005: 65).

Perhaps the most significant impact on communities is the increased burden posed by the dependents (both young and old) resulting from AIDS deaths. AIDS compromises the intergenerational contract that holds parents responsible for their children and expects children to return the favour when their parents age. Some social scientists have called this the 'intergenerational bargain' (Carmichael and Charles 1999 and Collard 1999 in Barnett and Whiteside 2006: 210). Moreover, those left behind are often not only affected by HIV and AIDS but could also be infected (Barnett and Whiteside 2006: 211). It is here that the community is expected to step in and 'adopt' the young and old into their care.

This increased burden of care, imposed on society as the productive members of society die and leave behind the young and the elderly, is often carried by the female members of society. The surviving mother, grandmother, aunt or other female relative is much more likely to look after orphans or the elderly than their male counterparts. It is also usually the eldest girl-child of the surviving offspring that takes responsibility for her younger (and older male) siblings (Marais 2005: 72; Monash and Snoad 2003).

AIDS orphans According to UNAIDS (2006), AIDS in South Africa has orphaned more than 1.2 million South African children – they are left to fend for themselves in a socio-political milieu that is already hugely burdened and extremely hostile.[8] In most cases these children are passed on to their network of relatives. It is here that the community is taking serious strain. Whilst African communities have typically embraced orphans into their midst, the sheer size of the orphan problem is eroding this sense of goodwill and compassion as a matter of necessity (Fröhlich 2008: 353).

Growing numbers of AIDS orphans also affect non-orphaned children. This comes as households within the community take on these orphans. The increased size of the family means that there are fewer resources available to the 'original' children of the household (Barnett and Whiteside 2006: 222).

Large numbers of orphans have also given rise to speculation about long-term state security and political instability. Their circumstances leave destitute children little choice but to live from hand-to-mouth. It is feared that this might make them reckless and cause them to disregard laws and norms, resulting in a breakdown of order (Barnett 2006: 299). These orphans are thought to constitute a lost generation who face little to no chance of rehabilitation back into society through education or employment. Although difficult to determine with accuracy, the effects of such a lost generation on society are bound to be significant.

Apart from the impact they have on society, orphans face a number of consequences as individuals. They are often socially excluded during the illness and death their parent(s) or otherwise shunned for fear that they too might be infected. They are also subjected to general neglect as the illness and subsequent death of a parent puts severe strain on resources and time available to educate and socialise children. As a result AIDS orphans are less likely to attend school and more likely to suffer depression. After the death of their parent(s), particularly girl orphans are vulnerable to sexual exploitation and abuse (Du Boisrouvray 2000: 165).

AIDS orphans are usually forced to grow up much faster than their non-orphaned counterparts. These changes may start as soon as the parent falls ill, when children are expected to care for their ailing elders. This also has serious psychological implications for children as they are confronted with the deteriorating health of

8 See Stein (2003) for a review of the impacts of HIV and AIDS on children and orphans.

their parent(s) (Marais 2005: 72). To add to their trauma, orphans could be passed on to old or infected caregivers. This means that these children could face a repeat of the trauma of illness and death and finally abandonment (Barnett and Whiteside 2006: 223).

The elderly Not only do those who die as a result of AIDS leave behind their children but also their parents who in their old age are suddenly without caregivers. Again, society and the state are expected to shoulder the responsibility. The effect of AIDS on the elderly is often neglected. Frequently construed as 'being on their way out anyway', they make a less attractive target for aid than the young who have their whole lives ahead of them.

Apart from losing their support structures both in terms of care and financial assistance when their children die of AIDS, the elderly are often also expected to take on their orphaned grandchildren (Barnett and Whiteside 2006: 232). In particular in rural societies, without their children the elderly are left to waste away in abject poverty. Without caregivers they often have no access to clean water and are forced to live without adequate shelter, clothing and food (Barnett and Whiteside 2006: 234).

Aggravating inequality AIDS has also had more subtle impacts on society. For one, it is widening social inequality by drawing stark lines between those that can afford treatment and those that cannot (Schneider and Moodie 2002: 8).

HIV and AIDS are also entrenching stereotypes already dangerously common in South Africa. Women are often seen as the carriers of AIDS and agents of contagion. As pregnant women are usually the first to notice that HIV has entered their lives, they are often seen as the ones who bring the disease. In South Africa AIDS is also riding on racial stereotypes, for instance portraying black people as having unusually large sexual appetites (Marais 2005: 15).

Economic impacts

Apart from leaving behind scores of dependents, given that AIDS fatalities occur mostly amongst the age cohort of the economically active, the AIDS epidemic has serious repercussions for agriculture, business and the economy as a whole.

Food supply On the most basic level, HIV and AIDS can limit supply of and access to food. De Waal and Whiteside (2003) argue that a 'new variant famine' is emerging as a result of AIDS. This famine is not the direct result of drought, but rather a consequence of reduced agricultural productivity. As AIDS illness and death leads to a loss of skills, labour, assets and implies less time for working the land, households are no longer able to sustain themselves through agriculture. This has serious implications for food security (De Waal and Whiteside 2003). Moreover, when farmers die prematurely their knowledge of agriculture dies with them before they have had the opportunity to pass on their skills to the next generation. Poor harvests mean poor nutrition, which leads to weakened immune systems that are more vulnerable to HIV infection (Schneider and Moodie 2002: 4). Finally, families may also lose out on the income that is generated through the sales of surplus crops (Barnett and Whiteside 2006: 238–61).

Industry AIDS can have even more profound effects on the economy, influencing the functioning of industry and large organisations. The United Nations Department of Economic and Social Affairs (UNDESA 2004: 53) suggest that HIV and AIDS affect firms through a number of processes. These include a reduction in the availability of workers due to AIDS deaths as well as the resultant loss of worker productivity as younger, less experienced workers replace those who have died. When skilled labourers are lost due to AIDS, the company may also lose some of the institutional knowledge it has accumulated over time. Organisations also risk losing profits due to increasing medical costs incurred in ensuring the wellbeing of their staff. Workers themselves will also face increased expenses due to increasing funerals and illness. This might also result in decreased morale amongst staff.

These effects can be placed into three categories: *direct costs* like health and life insurance, pension fund, recruitment, training and AIDS programmes, *indirect costs* like reduced productivity because of sick leave and reduced performance due to illness and *systemic costs* incurred through the cumulative impact of HIV and AIDS like reduction in overall staff morale, motivation and concentration and disruption of schedules (Barnett and Whiteside 2006: 274). Whilst these effects seem severe, the impact on the small business sector can be even harsher. Where an enterprise is run by only a few people AIDS illness and death can completely obliterate a business.

The economy AIDS not only impacts on the internal workings of industry, but also impacts on it from the outside. As the growing epidemic leads to increasing impoverishment of the general population, demand for goods may decline, slowing production (UNDESA 2004: 53). In a preliminary report Arndt and Lewis (2000) have suggested that, when compared to a no-AIDS scenario, by this year (2010) the South African economy would have lost 17 per cent of its GDP due to AIDS. Some of these losses can be attributed to a reduced workforce whilst per capita GDP has also experienced a decline.

These observations have led De Waal (2003) to propose assessing the effects of HIV and AIDS on the economy as a whole on two levels. The first takes issue with the direct costs of ill-health and premature death like spending on health care, funerals, the costs incurred as a result of reduced productivity and so on. The second category considers the consequences resulting from a changed demographic structure like a smaller working class and more dependents (De Waal 2003: 6). These changes have the potential to not only compromise a state's prospects for development but also to impair its ability to respond effectively to the epidemic, further escalating the crisis (Poku 2004: 47).

Political impacts

Good governance has become a central concept in the rhetoric around African progress and development. This can easily be deduced from, for example, the Commission for Africa's assertion that issues of bad governance lie at the heart of all of Africa's problems, or the New Partnership for Africa's Development's (NEPAD) assertion that 'democracy and good governance' are the key to poverty eradication and socio-economic development (Jones and Koffeld 2008: 97).

The impacts of HIV and AIDS on governance have not been well explored (Barnett and Whiteside 2006: 334). This is partly due to the long-wave nature of the epidemic, making it difficult to determine with certainty how the effects of HIV and AIDS will play out in the arena of politics. As a result much of the theory around political impact is still just that – theory, with a great reliance on scenario-building, educated guesses and speculation.

De Waal (2003: 11) suggests that decreased life expectancies due to AIDS will have two significant effects on governance: it compromises political participation and threatens to diminish the institutional capacity of a state. This means that HIV and AIDS both impede a government's ability to run itself and on a wider scale have serious implications for democracy.

Government The effects of HIV and AIDS on government are thought to play out in two ways: first through putting a greater demand on resources and reducing available funds and second on the institutional level through loss of staff. This affects the government's role as collector and spender of revenue as well as service provider and governing body (Barnett and Whiteside 2006: 319).

A drain on government resources and funding can be caused by a number of things. For instance, as HIV and AIDS take their toll on the economy, government revenue will decrease. This happens as GDP declines due to businesses' lost profits or as entire companies relocate to countries where AIDS is less prevalent. Moreover, the process of collecting revenue could itself be affected due to diminished institutional capacity (Barnett and Whiteside 2006: 323).

In particular, the South African health department is hit hard by the epidemic. Although according to Colvin (2008: 336) the available data on the effect of AIDS on the health care system is limited, AIDS does make increased demands on health services. The result is that the available resources are insufficient to provide and care for all who are ill (Colvin 2008: 344). This is perceived to be a great shortcoming of the state.

On the institutional level governments are affected by the loss of their staff and ruling elite. As older more experienced and well-networked staff die in their prime they are hastily replaced by their younger, inexperienced cadres. This places considerable strain on the system and in the long-term threatens to make administrations more criminalised, violent and prone to corruption. Parties could even begin to resemble their 'thuggish youth wings' (De Waal 2003: 15). The loss of senior political staff is not new to South Africa. By 2004 AIDS is thought to have claimed the lives of a Senior Presidential advisor, a sitting Cabinet Minister and a legislative back-bencher – all in the ruling party (Mattes and Manning 2004: 201).

Institutional capacity is further eroded as the South African epidemic is claiming a large number of public educators (Peltzer 2008: 103). Also, as education is an important channel for raising AIDS awareness and consciousness amongst younger people, this could further compound the issue (Peltzer 2008: 104).

The South African security sector is also hard-hit by HIV and AIDS. The loss of police members has serious repercussions for the maintenance of law and order, whilst loss of military personnel has broader implications for peacekeeping. There has been speculation that the South African National Defence Force (SANDF) is so weakened by AIDS that it will soon be too short-staffed to send troops on peacekeeping missions (Schneider and Moodie 2002: 6–7).

So far the discussion has focused on the effects of HIV and AIDS on government. However, government is also expected to react in a preventative and pre-emptive manner. This would include the establishment of AIDS institutions, inviting civil society and PWAs to participate in the policy process, establishing and maintaining accountability towards PWAs, maintaining transparency and responding quickly and effectively to issues, exhibiting sound and exemplary political leadership, the correct and effective use of law to protect PWAs, as well as a willingness and openness to discuss AIDS issues. A response of this scale makes further demands on government resources and staff. This means that HIV and AIDS affect government not only in terms of their direct consequences but also through managing and controlling the epidemic (Jones and Koffeld 2008: 102).

Democracy Some scholars have looked beyond the effects on government to investigate the possible effects of HIV and AIDS on democracy as a whole. A study by Strand et al. (2004) warns that AIDS could 'undermine South Africa's democratic project'. The study specifically investigates the effects of AIDS on the electoral process. It found that by hitting the economically active groups the hardest (and therefore also the politically active) AIDS has the potential to significantly diminish voting populations. Moreover, AIDS deaths are leading to a severe lack of skilled public servants that are necessary for the election process to run smoothly (Strand et al. 2004: 16).

Mattes and Manning (2004: 193) have added an economic consideration to the future of democracy, pointing out that wealthier states are more likely to and capable of sustaining democratic rule than poorer ones that might easily slip into authoritarian rule. As is apparent from the above discussion, AIDS undermines both poverty reduction and development goals, threatening the economic prosperity of a country.

Security In its most extensive sense, HIV and AIDS have significantly influenced how states think about security. The end of the Cold War has brought about a new definition of security that considers some non-violent threats to be as devastating to human welfare as violent threats. This new notion is known as human security (first formalised in the United Nations Development Programme's (UNDP) *Development Report* in 2004). The devastating toll that HIV and AIDS take on populations makes it a serious threat to human security (Hadingham 2000: 120). It threatens economic stability, food security, governance and political stability and is speculated to exacerbate crime and conflict (Fourie and Schönteich 2001). Consequently, Schneider and Moodie (2002: 3) have likened the impact of HIV and AIDS to prolonged armed conflict. As with an ongoing war it has the potential to compromise the state as a whole, on every conceivable level.

Conclusion

As this discussion has shown, the current state of the AIDS epidemic only presents the tip of the iceberg. Its effects are inherently difficult to measure, even harder to predict and therefore frequently understated. Insights into epidemiology and long-wave events put this against an even more troubling setting: this is an event that will not be over anytime soon. In fact, the worst is still to come. By the same token, knowledge of this creeping nature of the epidemic points to deeper implications for blame and accountability. Viewed against this reality it is clear that successive South African governments' slow responses to AIDS are a deeply troubling issue that is well worthy of investigation.

Chapter 3

Developing a Theory of Government AIDS Denial

The preceding chapters have already alluded to the maladies of inaction and failed intervention that have exacerbated the South African epidemic. In the early 1980s, when the first two AIDS deaths were recorded in South Africa, the apartheid government failed to acknowledge the risk HIV posed to the general population, presenting it as an affliction limited to the fringes of society. Their response to evidence that the epidemic was making a heterosexual transition followed a similar route as they continued to assure the white public they were not at risk as HIV affected mostly the black population. To their minds this eliminated the need for further government intervention. Towards the end of the 1980s government began to acknowledge the epidemic, publically announcing plans to counter it. However, these promises failed to translate into action, overshadowed by the liberation struggle.

The epidemic's slow, creeping start meant that the significance of the apartheid government's inadequate response only really became apparent a decade later. The clarity offered by hindsight makes arguments that the government was in a deliberate state of official denial at that time problematic. Government's largely rhetorical response and general inaction in the early stages of the epidemic could have simply been a matter of not knowing any better. Nonetheless, these initial elements of denial point towards the beginning of a trend that would become ever more pronounced as the epidemic intensified, escalating to a point where official denial finally reached the public consciousness during Mbeki's two administrations.

South Africa's peaceful transition to democracy eventually led to more tangible plans to counter AIDS. In 1992 the National AIDS Convention of South Africa (NACOSA) was established and South Africa's first National AIDS Plan (NAP) was conceived in 1994. Although commended as an impeccable document, the NAP was poorly implemented and the AIDS issue was again denied priority status. In this case, the new democratic dispensation's failure to implement an effective response to the epidemic could have been more a matter of institutional incapacity than deliberate attempts at denial. But that HIV infection spread rampantly at this time had serious implications for subsequent leadership. Moreover, as is discussed later in this book, denying a pressing issue the attention it deserves could in some cases be a deliberate means of avoiding the awkward admission of being incapable of appropriately responding to the situation.

What must be kept in mind is that South African governments' early failures to respond adequately to the epidemic meant that infection spread almost exponentially since the first cases of AIDS were reported in 1982. And yet it was really only once ARVs became an affordable treatment option in the mid-1990s that government inaction became an obvious concern. With the correct response to the epidemic now undeniably clear, government's failure could no longer be excused as a symptom of an uninformed, ineffective or otherwise distracted bureaucracy. Suddenly official lethargy was dubbed 'denial' and public outcry reached a shrill crescendo. There is no doubt that Mbeki's term of office marked an unprecedented concentration of controversy and denialism and that it was largely deserving of this criticism. But the unique nature of the epidemic suggests that blame cannot be exclusively allocated to his inaction and neither then should suspicions and accusations of official denial be confined to his governments.

As this chapter will show, the increase in HIV prevalence and morbidity that significantly contributed to the furore around the Mbeki governments' dealings with the epidemic had been brewing long before he came to power. Drawing on existing government critique and building on our earlier discussion of long-wave events, this chapter proposes a theory of denial that incorporates all government action (and therefore the possibility of inaction and denial) since the first two South African AIDS cases were publicised in 1982. The discussion then turns its attention to finding an appropriate tool that would facilitate closer investigation of this theory of government denial. London School of Economics (LSE) academic Stanley Cohen's typology of official denial is discussed as the most appropriate means to both identify and analyse possible instances of government AIDS denial.

Of hope and hopelessness: ARVs and government reluctance

The development and affordability of ARVs represents a significant watershed in South Africa's AIDS story. Effectively, ARVs redefined the AIDS problem, transforming a death sentence into a manageable chronic condition. However, at the time the South African government seemed less than thrilled with this new development and resorted to an intriguing array of arguments to delay rollout by over a decade.

The dazzling new sense of hope offered by treatment cast a new light on government's hopelessness. The availability of an effective treatment meant that for the first time government's failure to respond adequately to the epidemic became painfully obvious, as official inaction could no longer be put down to a lack of adequate treatment options. The South African government was subjected to unprecedented scrutiny and former President Mbeki found himself at the centre of much outrage. It seemed quite logical that his contestation of AIDS science and his government's refusal to make ARVs readily and cheaply available were almost entirely to blame for the scale of the South African AIDS epidemic. The media, civil society and the scientific community appeared to be unequivocal on the matter – were it not for Mbeki and his quack Ministers of Health, South Africa would have escaped the worst impacts of the AIDS epidemic.

ARVs enter the scene

Although research into treatment options commenced almost immediately after the HI virus was identified in the early 1980s, this search was marred by a great deal of pessimism, underpinned by the belief that retroviruses were fundamentally untreatable. In 1987 this notion was proved wrong when azidothymidine (also known as zidovudene or AZT) was granted approval by the US Food and Drug Administration (FDA) and became the first anti-retroviral treatment for AIDS (Nelson 2006: 466). AZT (a nucleoside thymidine analogue) had a remarkable initial success rate. But enthusiasm for AZT soon waned when it became apparent that the HI virus quickly developed a resistance to AZT. The drug has also had a number of unwanted side effects (Kallings 2008: 223).

Nonetheless, this breakthrough paved the way for further research. Consequently, the early 1990s saw a significant diversification of the HIV drug repertoire, including the development of a number of additional nucleoside analogues as well as non-nucleoside inhibitors of reverse transcriptase, protease inhibitors and entry inhibitors (Kallings 2008: 223). In 1994 it was discovered that AZT reduced the risk of vertical MTCT. This meant that the likelihood of a foetus contracting HIV from its mother could be significantly reduced. In 1999 a clinical trial in Uganda proved the effectiveness of another MTCT prevention drug – Nevirapine. Although fulfilling essentially the same function as AZT, Nevirapine is substantially cheaper and easier to administer (Nattrass 2007: 62).

However, it was only in 1996 when a particular combination treatment of three AIDS drugs was introduced that HIV treatment became viable at scale. What became known as 'highly active anti-retroviral therapy' (HAART) significantly reduced the risk of resistance and promised to have unprecedented long-term efficacy (Kallings 2008: 223).[1] From there on it was only a matter of time until the process of taking HAART was simplified and many of its unpleasant and dangerous side effects were eliminated (Kallings 2008: 223).

Collectively these developments signified a massive breakthrough. Through correct administration ARVs can significantly extend the lives of those suffering from AIDS, as well as improve their quality of life (Cameron 2000: 10). In effect AIDS became a manageable chronic disease and as Schneider and Moodie (2002: 4) have pointed out ever since, the international community has been fully capable of making the treatment available.

---

1 HAART is any anti-retroviral regimen that can suppress HIV for many years. It usually involves the use of two reverse transcriptase inhibitors and one protease inhibitor (Barnett and Whiteside 2006: 47).

South African reluctance

Whilst some states embraced this new opportunity to radically reduce or at least to buffer the devastating effects of HIV and AIDS and began their ARV rollout as soon as the drug was made available, South Africa's reaction was underscored by a lethargy that has been widely criticised.

To highlight the positive impact of achieving early ARV rollout, South Africa's response can be contrasted to that of Brazil. Whilst the two developing, middle-income countries share many similarities (like racial diversity, colonial legacies, income inequality and a high Gini coefficient) they chose to respond very differently to HIV and AIDS. In 1991 the Brazilian government began providing AZT to all patients with clinical AIDS. In 1996 the Brazilian Congress passed legislation that required the public healthcare system to provide all necessary medications for AIDS patients; this included the provision of HAART (Gauri and Lieberman 2006: 55). For Brazil this intervention has resulted in a significant reduction in the prevalence and impact of AIDS. In South Africa, on the other hand, ARVs remained unavailable to the general public until 2002/3 (and then only very slowly after that). The many detours the government took to rollout cost the country dearly.

As noted in Chapter 6, determined to find an 'African solution' for the AIDS problem, in 1997 the South African government enthusiastically pushed for approval of the locally developed drug, Virodene. Heralded by scientists from the University of Pretoria as a new miracle cure for AIDS, Virodene failed to pass even the most elementary biological and animal experimentation and was declared unfit for testing on humans (Schneider and Stein 2001: 728). In the following year the government announced that it would not provide AZT for the prevention of MTCT. This would not be cost-effective, they argued, in spite of a growing number of studies showing that the long-term economic benefits of introducing AZT by far outweighed its immediate costs.

When AZT was made available more cheaply, following a fierce battle with pharmaceutical companies over patents, the government stopped arguing finance and started contesting science, expressing doubts about the efficacy of AZT and claiming that it was toxic. That AZT was endorsed both by South Africa's Medical Control Council as well as the US FDA and CDC had little impact on the government.

Relief finally came in 2002 when a South African Constitutional Court ruling *forced* the government to issue Nevirapine for MTCTP. HAART was only made available the following year. Even then rollout was frustratingly slow. More than a decade after ARVs became an affordable treatment option, rollout continued to be hopelessly lethargic. By December 2007, according to the WHO (2008: 120), only 28 per cent of the population in need of ARVs was receiving treatment. In neighbouring Botswana, 79 per cent of those in need received ARVs. In Namibia rollout reached 88 per cent. There is wide consensus that treatment rollout should never have been delayed in this manner.

Accusations of government denial begin to take shape

Engaging in large-scale ARV rollout is certainly a formidable task for any developing country. However this slow response could not merely have been a matter of insufficient resources. At the time South Africa had considerably more funding at its disposal than other African states (many of which conducted far more effective AIDS campaigns) (Nattrass 2004: 29). In fact, South Africa has had adequate funding to ensure a universally accessible package of HIV prevention, care and support, including education and anti-retroviral therapy to HIV-positive pregnant women (Schneider and Stein 2001: 724). Moreover, there is a strong case to be made that providing HAART to all people with AIDS would make better financial sense than doing nothing and letting them die (Nattrass 2005). This assessment is based purely on monetary considerations pertaining to healthcare and does not include other less quantifiable (particularly moral) arguments in favour of HAART like fewer orphans, improved quality of life or reduced strain on the economy that would further sway the argument in favour of ARV rollout.

Given the effectiveness of ARVs, coupled with the evidence that there was in fact money available to provide this treatment, it became clear that the government itself became the main obstacle to treatment rollout. Many critics now pointed to government's inefficacy. In a recent study, Chigwedere et al. (2008) accuse the South African government of acting as 'a major obstacle' in providing medication to people living with the HI virus. They have used modelling to calculate the lives that were lost through government's failure to initiate a 'feasible and timely' ARV treatment programme. According to their calculations, in the period between 2000 and 2005 at least 330,000 lives could have been saved had the government acted appropriately. This has led to repeated calls for an AIDS-specific Truth and Reconciliation Commission (TRC) that would investigate these unnecessary deaths and hold the government accountable.[2]

Kallings (2008: 224) has similarly remarked that in South Africa the cost of treatment is no longer the greatest obstacle to rollout; during the tenure of Thabo Mbeki the greatest obstacle was the lack of political will, along with a lack of healthcare infrastructure. UN Special Envoy for HIV and AIDS in Africa, Stephen Lewis (2006: 3), accused the government of being 'obtuse, dilatory and negligent' about rollout and questioned the government's role as a compassionate state. Nattrass (2004: 41) has called it a 'sorry tale of missed opportunities, inadequate analysis, bureaucratic failure and political mismanagement'. According to Barnett and Whiteside (2006: 317) 'the most extreme manifestation of government's inability to respond has been in South Africa'. Ndinga-Muvumba and Scanlon (2006: 18) have more subtly remarked that local governments in South Africa are yet to comprehend the full impact of AIDS on society as well as respond adequately to the epidemic, and Gaurie and Liebermann (2006: 47) have called the South African government a 'laggard'.

---

2 See Karrim (2009) as well as *The Lancet* (2006).

But the South African government's failure to respond with the required sense of urgency pointed to something more grave and deep-seeded than lethargy and mismanagement. A number of other controversies accompanied government's contestation of ARVs:

- Thabo Mbeki's stated beliefs that HIV could not be the cause of AIDS.
- The then Minister of Health's preference for vitamins and vegetables to treat AIDS, rather than ARVs (Geffen 2006; McGregor 2009; Thom 2009).
- Mbeki's claims that poverty and crime are the biggest killers in South Africa; and
- The Mbeki government's argument that AIDS is part of a neo-colonialist plot devised by Westerners (pharmaceutical companies in particular) to continue exploiting Africa and to dehumanise its people (Wang 2008).

This has led many to emphasise denial as an underlying motive for government's failure to implement adequate treatment and prevention programmes. Schneider and Moodie (2002: 5) have argued that HIV and AIDS are 'too often greeted with complacency and denial by local officials'. Van Niekerk (2001: 149) more explicitly argues that the South African government is in a 'state of denial'. Geffen (2006: 2) has similarly suggested that instead of a lack of resources being the government's biggest obstacle, a state-sponsored pseudo-science has stood in the way of effective treatment action. Kalichman (2009: 127) has noted that 'denialism has plagued South Africa nearly as badly as the epidemic itself'. Other references to denial have been more subtle and include those made by Altman (2006), Barnett, Prins and Whiteside (2005: 21) as well as Marais (2005: 15).

However, in the heat of government's refusals to provide ARVs and media coverage of the accompanying scandals at the time, these accusations of denial seem to be levelled almost exclusively at Mbeki's governments (1999–2004; 2004–08). When viewed against the long-wave nature of the epidemic these allegations raise concerns regarding accountability. Less than a year after Mbeki became President, in 2000, already 3,559,585 South Africans were HIV-positive (Dorrington et al. 2006: 24). It follows that denial by successive Mbeki administrations cannot account for the current scale of the South African AIDS epidemic in its entirety. Moreover, whilst ARVs introduced a revolutionary and hugely effective means of responding to the epidemic, ARVs are only a reactive measure. A comprehensive plan would have to be both proactive in terms of prevention as well as reactive in terms of treatment. Such proactive responses were available long before ARVs were developed and limited only by the strategic and resource allocation skills of officials.

One can thus argue that the South African government could and should have responded to HIV and AIDS with greater urgency long before the development of ARVs in the 1990s. An effective intervention (pre-ARVs) would have included prevention programmes, AIDS awareness and education campaigns, counselling and medical support for the sick. Some critics have included this in their considerations. Heywood (2004: 2) has suggested that the transition to democracy and consequent social reconstruction have at times been 'accompanied by attempts to ignore, hide and marginalise the advance of the HIV and AIDS epidemic'. Furlong and Ball (2005: 127) suggest that it is a widely held view that the pre-1994 apartheid government, 'hidebound by Puritanism and racism, ignored or at best paid lip service to the AIDS threat'. Grundlingh (2001) also indicates that the apartheid administrations' strategy to downplay the severity of the disease and its potential to spread only compounded HIV and AIDS.

This evidence necessitates an investigation into government action that goes beyond the much debated, publicised and scrutinised responses of the Mbeki governments. In light of the drawn-out nature of the epidemic it becomes necessary to investigate whether successive governments could have been at least in part responsible for the current state of the epidemic. By the same reasoning, if denial is considered a driving factor for the Mbeki governments' inaction, then continued inaction preceding Mbeki could point to a history of official denial.

Reconsidering blame and denial in a long-wave event

Increased media attention to the issue of AIDS may make the epidemic appear to be the result largely of mismanagement by the Mbeki governments. However the unique characteristics of the epidemic point to a more complex relationship between accountability, blame and denial. When Mbeki came to power in 1999 the situation he inherited was already overwhelming. This suggests two things: that the current extent of the epidemic can be traced back to some extent to mismanagement or neglect by the Mandela and apartheid governments and, that the effects of continued mismanagement and neglect at present will only really be felt in five to ten years' time. Here our earlier discussion (Chapter 2) of epidemic curves and long-wave events and their implications for statistics regarding the South African epidemic allows for a clearer illustration of the situation.[3]

As Figure 3.1 shows, by 2000, soon after Mbeki's inauguration as President, 302,790 South Africans had already died of AIDS since 1982. Although these deaths were drawing attention to the growing epidemic, a much larger crisis was looming. Whilst these deaths were suggesting the situation required some urgency, what was not yet obvious was the latent illness of the 3,559,585 HIV infections in 2000 (indicated by the dotted arrow). As these people were not yet sick, the impact of their HIV infection went largely unnoticed. Without medical intervention in the form of ARVs these infections would become increasingly noticeable over the next ten years as the some 3.5 million HIV-positive people gradually develop AIDS and die. By 2004, when Mbeki commenced his second term in office, the

3 However, keep in mind that this data is largely conjectural. It is drawn from the study by Dorrington et al. (2006) and serves to explain, at least in principle, how the long-wave nature of AIDS complicates issues of blame and accountability.

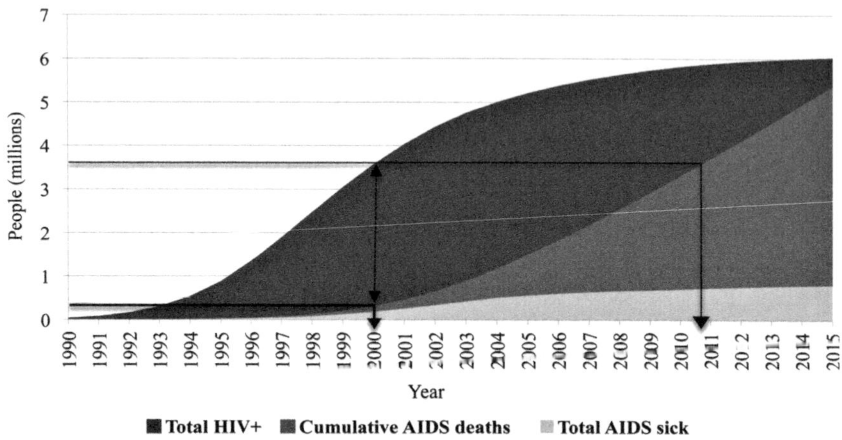

Figure 3.1 The South African epidemic as a long-wave event
Source: Data from Dorrington et al. (2006: 21).

total number of AIDS deaths had increased nearly five-fold from 2000, to close to 1.5 million. Without the critical intervention of ARVs it would take until mid-2010 for all the persons that were HIV-positive when Mbeki first assumed office in 1999 to have fallen ill with AIDS.

Whilst this sketches a rather morbid picture it also provides a fresh perspective on issues of responsibility and accountability. That some 3.5 million people were already HIV-positive when Mbeki assumed office was not within the control of his government. Whilst the escalating AIDS death toll may have appeared to be the result solely of both Mbeki governments' failure to roll out ARVs, the deaths that unfolded under Mbeki's rule were the consequence of infections that occurred under the leadership of his predecessors during the two previous decades. Mbeki inherited a country in which 3.5 million people would die within the next ten years, if no action were taken. In many ways he commenced his presidency sitting on a ticking time bomb.

However, as De Waal (2002: 3) cautions, whilst the first two waves of HIV and AIDS – infection, illness (and death) – are already manifest in South Africa, there is 'nothing inevitable' about the third wave – impact. Instead he argues that through correct political action and by bringing an end to the 'complacency and self-inflicted ignorance' that has characterised government response in the last two decades, the third 'impact' wave can be buffered and managed effectively. This raises an important point: whilst the Mbeki government cannot be blamed for the HIV infections it inherited, it can be held accountable for its failure to respond adequately and timely, thus failing to prevent unnecessary deaths and broader impacts. This is a particularly emotive issue, as the means to provide life-saving treatment were there – only the political will was lacking, underwritten to some extent by denial. Moreover, the Mbeki government can (as ARVs have a cumulative prevention effect) to some extent also be held accountable for many of the HIV infections that occurred on its watch.

Government action and inaction prior to Mbeki provide an additional perspective. Figure 3.2 allows for a closer look at the ten years preceding Mbeki's first term as President. In 1993, as the country was preparing for democratisation, the epidemic was on the rise: already 301,999 people were HIV-positive (indicated by the grey arrow). Barely visible on the graph at this stage are the 4,778 cumulative AIDS deaths and the 3,787 people sick with AIDS at that stage (Dorrington et al. 2006: 21). As most of the HIV-positive people were not yet sick, their infection was not all that visible as their illness still had no real effect on the community,

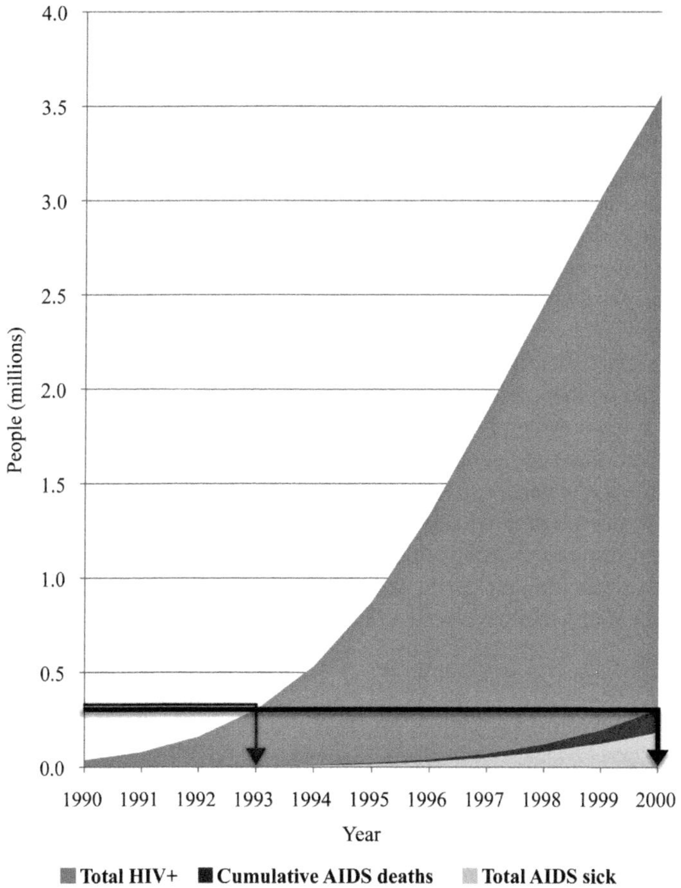

Figure 3.2 A closer look at accountability in the South African epidemic
Source: Data from Dorrington et al. (2006).

the economy or politics. At this time, leaders were either truly oblivious to the imminent epidemic, or it was relatively easy for them to give priority to different political issues (especially given the volatility of the political situation during the transition to democracy).

The full impact of the HIV infections in 1993 would only be felt once these people fell ill (and most likely died). This only really started to happen by 2000, just after Mbeki became Head of State (indicated by the black arrow). What the graph illustrates even more effectively is the number of additional HIV infections that occurred between 1993 and 2000. Had the government taken the necessary preventative steps around 1993, HIV infection might not have risen to 3,559,585 by 2000 and the Mbeki government would not have faced the death toll that it did. Brazil and Thailand both achieved significant success in curbing the AIDS epidemic by means of timely and effective intervention at similar phases of their epidemics (Gauri and Lieberman 2006; UNDP 2004).

This line of argument can be taken even further back. To account for the infections in 1993, events a decade prior should be assessed. This would take the analysis back to the very early years of AIDS in South Africa. Again the argument applies that had appropriate preventative action been taken then, there would not have been 301,999 HIV infections by 1993. Instead, in the period directly after the first two AIDS deaths were recorded in 1982, the apartheid government assured the white public that they were not at risk as the disease appeared to be limited to gay men, prostitutes, intravenous drug users and later the general black population. As these risk groups were held in great disdain by the government and the apartheid ethos effectively justified the continued abuse of their human rights, this conveniently eliminated the need for further government intervention. Whether government had any real inkling of the scientific truth about HIV at that time is unknown and this possibility of their ignorance does taint arguments around government denial during this time.

Regardless, the persistent and unchecked growth of the epidemic (both before and after ARVs became widely available) suggests a rich history of inadequate government response that has not been limited to the Mbeki governments. Indeed, if statistics are anything to go by, policies that were introduced since the 1980s to combat HIV and AIDS have been a dismal failure.

Formulating an AIDS denial 'hypothesis'

Given that the history of inadequate government responses can be traced back to the very first recorded AIDS deaths in South Africa, suggestions that the post-apartheid governments (and Mbeki in particular) have been in a state of denial over the HIV epidemic cannot by themselves account for the extent of the current epidemic. It is therefore quite likely that, as Furlong and Ball (2005: 129) have suggested, whilst there was denial in the post-1994 governments, there was also 'much denial' of HIV and AIDS amongst officials of the apartheid governments.

Clearly, instances of official neglect have preceded the governments of Thabo Mbeki. To which extent this can be considered a consequence of government denial is at this point unclear.

The discussion thus far points to a hypothesis of sorts: that South African governments have been in a state of denial over the HIV epidemic long before Mbeki's controversial tenure. Investigating this theory of denial requires a thorough assessment of successive governments' dealings with the epidemic since 1982 in order to establish two things: whether there have indeed been serious cases of government denial, and if so, if they were frequent enough to warrant the claim that this has been a 'continued state of denial'. That said, denial remains a highly abstract concept that is exceedingly difficult to prove. Any further investigation into government denial therefore necessitates both a thorough clarification of denial as well as an investigation into means for measuring denial.

Unpacking denial

South Africa certainly is not the only country to have responded to AIDS with denial. According to De Waal (2006: 11) the whole African continent must be reeling 'in a state of collective denial'. Although there is a more or less general acknowledgement of the epidemic, most African states have done little to deal with its actual consequences (De Waal 2006: 13). It would appear that government denial of AIDS is not an unusual response (Heywood 2004: 6). Officials in states across the world have struggled with HIV and AIDS denial since the 1980s. As Kallings (2008: 218) has argued, 'the subject of AIDS is emotionally and politically charged, and denial has frequently prevented rational counter-measures'. However, whereas official (government) denial of AIDS has been eroded and eventually negated by civil rights movements in most other countries, in South Africa it appears to have persisted (Heywood 2004: 7).

Government denial can have serious implications for a country, many of which are ultimately detrimental to the government itself. For one, it is a formidable obstruction to both the effective response to the AIDS epidemic as well as development overall. The development challenges for Africa are often grossly misunderstood because the crippling effect of AIDS is poorly understood (McPherson, Hoover and Snodgrass 2000: 10). Acknowledgement of the epidemic is therefore not only in the best interest of those infected and affected by HIV and AIDS, but also beneficial to the general population as well as the government.

Denialism vs. denial

Whilst the two terms are often used interchangeably, there is a critical difference between *denial of AIDS* and *AIDS denialism*. *AIDS denialism* is a view commonly held by AIDS dissidents. These dissident groups are typically characterised by an outright defiance for the medical field and therefore actively oppose scientific consensus on AIDS.[4] *Denial of AIDS* on the other hand extends beyond appeals made to the science of AIDS. Essentially, *denial of AIDS* would include instances of *AIDS denialism* as well as other attempts at disavowing issues relating to the epidemic. Arguing for instance that HIV is limited to homosexuals or prostitutes, or that there is insufficient funding available for treatment when in fact the government's AIDS budget allows for it, would be considered *denial of AIDS* rather than *AIDS denialism*. It is this wider, more inclusive definition of AIDS denial that underpins our study. By investigating denial as a whole, we can cast our net wider to consider more nuanced government responses that have gone beyond contesting the science of HIV and AIDS. The scope of our examination in this book therefore extends beyond the ambit of AIDS denialism and seeks to understand the role of denial in general in successive South African governments' responses. Thus it is in the interest of clarity for the discussion here that both *AIDS denialism* and *denial of AIDS* are conceptually clarified.

AIDS denialism Critique and dissidence regarding the science of AIDS was not unusual or even unexpected in the early 1980s when relatively little was known about AIDS pathogenesis (Nattrass 2007: 24). However, as knowledge and understanding of AIDS and its treatments deepened, many dissidents were swayed by the scientific evidence (amongst these were Joseph Sonnabend and Udo Schülenk). In contrast to these 'persuaded' dissidents, those who choose to continue their defiance of the mainstream AIDS science have become more popularly known as AIDS denialists (Nattrass 2007: 25). This transition in labels for dissidents is consistent with Cohen's observation that in order for something to be correctly termed 'denial' there must be an ultimate truth against which the denial becomes obvious (Cohen 2001: 6). There is now an abundance of incontestable scientific evidence vouching for the existence of HIV and AIDS, proving beyond all doubt that HIV causes AIDS. This is simply the reality, and the contestation of these facts can no longer be considered as mere scepticism or dissidence; rather, it is denial in its truest sense.

AIDS denialists are characterised by an outright defiance of the medical and scientific field and therefore actively oppose scientific consensus on AIDS.[5] Nattrass (2007: 22–3) distinguishes between two groups within the AIDS denialist community. The first argues that HIV and AIDS do not exist. This includes the notorious Perth Group in Australia. The second accepts the existence of HIV but instead considers it a non-threat. Instead they believe that AIDS deaths are really only a result of a number of precipitating conditions, including malnutrition,

4 See for example Duesberg (1991), Duesberg and Rasnick (1998) and The Perth Group (2008).

5 See for example Duesberg (1991), Duesberg and Rasnick (1998) and the Perth Group (2008).

narcotics and anti-retroviral therapies themselves. This group typically follows Peter Duesberg, a molecular biologist at the University of California.

Through their active campaigning, particularly on the Internet, the denialists have gained a surprising amount of support. Amongst their most influential supporters have been the likes of Thabo Mbeki. The former South African President's fascination with AIDS denialism became public when he began questioning AIDS statistics and the safety of ARVs in 1999. This, some critics lamented, gave new life to the denialist movement that at the time was losing its relevance (Nattrass 2007: 33). Although Mbeki's office now claims that he never categorically denied that HIV causes AIDS (in effect denying the denialism), Mbeki's statements in September 2000 (Agence France Press 2000) that a virus cannot cause a syndrome and that therefore HIV cannot cause AIDS is a matter of public record. Mbeki has questioned the link sufficiently to undermine South Africa's progress in the fight against AIDS and to cast considerable doubt on his faith in science.

On the whole, South Africa has had a longstanding affair with AIDS denialism. Examples include former Minister of Health Tshabalala-Msimang's endorsement of vitamins and vegetables to treat HIV (not as complementary but rather as alternatives to ARVs), government's refusal to roll out ARVs based on the argument that AZT is in fact toxic, refusing mainstream scientific assessments of the drug Virodene and attempting to approve it anyway (Cullinan and Thom 2009). These cases of denialism will be discussed in greater detail in the following chapters.

Denial of AIDS Whilst AIDS denialism characterised the Mbeki governments' reactions to the epidemic, prior government inaction is more likely to have been the result of other forms of denial that were not necessarily directed at the science of the epidemic. This included, for instance, arguing that only homosexuals or commercial sex workers carry the disease. In order to investigate possibilities of government denial more thoroughly, a broader conceptualisation of denial is required.

LSE scholar Stanley Cohen has grappled extensively with denial and offers a very broad and general definition of it (Cohen 2001: 1):

> People, organizations, governments or whole societies are presented with information that is too disturbing, threatening or anomalous to be fully absorbed or openly acknowledged. The information is therefore somehow repressed, disavowed, pushed aside or reinterpreted. Or else the information 'registers' well enough, but its implications – cognitive, emotional or moral – are evaded, neutralized or rationalized.

HIV and AIDS are particularly likely to foster denial. The disease forces the disclosure of sexual behaviour and is an unwelcome intruder into the private sphere. This often causes individuals to deny their own illness or the risks they may face in contracting it, especially through sex. HIV also lays bare other vulnerabilities and preys on social inequalities. HIV is a free-riding infection that targets weakened immune systems. This ties in closely with issues of poverty and in the South African case poverty in turn relates to issues of race. Poor healthcare and desperate conditions also contribute to the rampant spread of STIs (further compounded by the migrant labour system). Sexually transmitted infections (STIs), in particular those causing genital ulcering, significantly increase the chances of acquiring HIV, as well as of transmitting it (Corey et al. 2004). Overall, this makes acknowledging and addressing HIV and AIDS a sensitive and uncomfortable task – both for individuals and government officials.

Taboo and denial often feed off each other (Altman 2006: 134). Whilst AIDS denial is aimed at the illness itself ('I do not have AIDS') denial can also be directed at the epidemic in general ('there is no epidemic'), as well as its potential ('it will never get that bad…'). However, reasons for government denial go well beyond mere awkwardness. Government denial is most commonly used to evade responsibility. According to Nepal (2007: 135–6) AIDS denial has been a significant cause of the 'low, slow, and fragmented responses' of Asian officials. Nepal's (2007: 134–6) assessment of Asian government's mismanagement of the epidemic effectively illustrates the many forms of denial (including AIDS denialism) that officials can resort to in order to escape accountability. These include:

- Contesting AIDS science (dissidence or denialism).
- Arguing that AIDS is a foreigners' disease and therefore does not pose a considerable threat to locals.
- Proposing that society is inherently moral and will abstain from deviant behaviour that could expose them to the virus.
- Suggesting that because the virus only affects deviant members of society, the majority of morally uncorrupted citizens are insulated anyway.
- Condemning those that have HIV because they have brought it upon themselves with their morally deviant behaviour.
- Keeping statistics hidden and confidential; and
- Disagreeing over the scale of the epidemic and questioning the accuracy of estimates like those from UNAIDS.

Similar tactics can be observed in South African governments' responses to the epidemic. However, as our investigation will consider nearly three decades of government action and inaction, investigating allegations of South African government denial requires a typology of official denial that can be applied repeatedly and consistently in order to highlight possible instances of denial. The search for an appropriate tool thus commences with a review of the existing literature on government AIDS denial. Investigating government denial requires a sound understanding of the mechanisms of denial. To this end, a review of the literature of denial is appropriate.

A review of existing literature on denial

The first person to really grapple extensively with issues of denial was Sigmund Freud.[6] As he approached the issue from a psychoanalytical vantage point, Freud's discussions of denial and repression were restricted to the individual. Theories of denial have since then evolved into a very broad field that has found wide appeal across a number of disciplines. It has featured particularly frequently in discussions around racism or ethnic tensions. In particular, Holocaust denial has often drawn on theories around denial.[7] Within his context, theories of denial have often been used to explain particular behaviour. For instance, Van Dijk (1992) has used denial as a means to better understand racism in the press whilst Cohan (2002) discussed the influence denial had in the Enron scandal. Denial also frequents discussions of environmental issues.[8]

However, it is the application of theories of denial within the discipline of Politics and more specifically to government responses in the face of controversies that is of real interest in this study. Again, here denial is most frequently used as a theory that might offer an explanation for certain behaviour or actions. Beyrer (2003) for instance argues that denial is often a key motivator in government's mishandling of public health threats. Jalusic and Dedic (2008) have argued that Slovenian officials have resorted to denial after being accused of removing Serbian, Croatian and Bosnian residents from the registry of citizens and listing them instead as aliens.

Thus far, perhaps the most dynamic assessment of government denial as been conducted by LSE scholar Stanley Cohen. Writing extensively on official denial as a response to human rights abuse claims, in 1996 Cohen devised a typology of denial against which government responses can be measured. In 2001 Cohen refined this typology and broadened its application to extend beyond human rights disputes. His modified typology is a highly effective means of analysing government rhetoric to highlight elements of official denial. The typology distinguishes between three broad categories of government denial: classic official denial, counter offensive denial (pointing out the shortfalls of the initial accusers as a means to discredit them) and partial acknowledgement (in which the event is not entirely denied, but there is no recourse). Classic official denial is again subdivided into three categories: literal denial (arguing that an event did not occur), interpretive denial (challenging the existing definition of the event with an alternative version) or implicatory denial (attempting to pass the event off as being justified).

Cohen's typology has found appeal with a number of analysts. Welch (2003) has used it to suggest that officials were largely in denial about human rights abuses

6 Although Freud used the term 'Verleugnung', which is more akin to disavowal than denial.

7 For instance, see Bischoping (1997), Lasson (2007) and McKinnon (2007).

8 Amongst others, Bower (1997) and Markowitz and Rosner (2003) discuss issues of pollution and the environment with reference to denial.

during the war on terror, whilst Hegarty (2004) incorporated the typology into an assessment of the official responses to Bloody Sunday. Zerouali (1999) used Cohen's typology to assess official denial in response to the Algerian Massacres.[9]

Specifically within the context of AIDS, denial has also been widely covered. In this case, however, literature dealing specifically with the denial of mainstream science (AIDS denialism) dominates the field. These include writings by the dissidents themselves (Duesberg 1991; Duesberg and Rasnick 1998; the Perth Group 2008) as well as the many criticisms and discussions of these denialist positions (Heywood 2004; Nattrass 2007). Other literature dealing with AIDS denial considers the role of denial in the AIDS epidemic in general (Altman 2006; Barnett 2006), whilst authors like Barnett and Whiteside (2006: 6) as well as De Waal (2006: 12) have offered explanations for this denial. Nepal (2007) for instance has constructed a very insightful assessment of AIDS denial in Asia.

Literature relating specifically to South African cases of government denial can be divided into roughly two categories: those that provide a (sometimes historical) overview of official denial in the South African AIDS epidemic (Furlong and Ball 2005; Grundlingh 2001; Heywood 2004) and those that attempt to explain this denial by suggesting motives and other agendas (Fassin 2002; Geffen 2006; Schneider and Marais 2005; Wang 2008). However, these accounts are for the larger part restricted to commentaries and none of these authors have made denial their main focus. Particularly President Thabo Mbeki has at times been the centre of debate in this issue, with two recent works (Gevisser 2007; Roberts 2007) debating the former President's role in the AIDS epidemic. It is within this broader scope of denial of AIDS and more specifically the allegations of successive South African governments' denial that this book proceeds.

Investigating government denial

Even with a sound grasp of denial, allegations of government denial are still not easily proven. Government denial is most frequently found in rhetoric – the communication resulting between key figures within a government and the media, the government's critics and supporters, as well as the general public (Cohen 2001: 4, 102). It follows that evidence of denial is seldom found in policy or other official documentation but rather in the public relations material of a government like speeches and media reports. Searching for signs of denial therefore requires analysing the rhetoric or communications of key policy makers, which in this case would include the Minister of Health, other officials within the Department of Health, as well as the President and other statements issued by government.

Accurately investigating government denial thus requires a tool that would facilitate careful assessment of policy makers' rhetoric when dealing with HIV and AIDS. Stanley Cohen's (2001) typology of official denial is well-suited for this

9 Zerouali, however, used Cohen's 1996 typology.

purpose. Through application of Cohen's typology, government responses can be analysed, classified and mapped against a continuum in order to achieve a sound understanding of the extent and severity of denial that may have been invoked in the South African official response to HIV and AIDS. This reveals further insight into the motivations and mechanisms of government denial.

Contextualising official denial

However, before applying Cohen's typology of official denial to South African government action, it is useful to first consider the nature of denial and how official denial relates to it. Cohen has identified six determining and underlying facets of denial. They are the *psychology* of denial (why is there denial?), the *content* of denial (what is being denied?), the *organisation* of denial (is it one person, a state or a community?), the *time* of denial (is it historic or contemporary?), the *agents* of denial (is the denying organisation the victim, perpetrator or observer?) and finally, the *space and place* of denial. These basic determinants of denial allow for a more precise delimitation of the alleged government denial that this study sets out to investigate.

Essentially, the *psychology* of denial grapples with the question: why is there denial? Cohen offers three possible explanations. The first considers that the suspected statement of denial is in fact the truth – that nothing happened, or that if it did, nothing is known by the agent (person or organisation) doing the denying. A second explanation considers that something did happen and that the agent denying it is aware of the incident. In such a case, the statement of denial would be 'deliberate, intentional and conscious' (Cohen 2001: 4). If it is an individual doing the denying, then it is considered a lie or concealment and if it is proposed by an institution, then it is referred to as propaganda, whitewash, spin, fraud, cover-up or disinformation (Cohen 2001: 4). Political denial, being 'cynical, calculated and transparent' would therefore be considered part of this deliberate type of denial (Cohen 2001: 6).

But denial can also be the result of a much less conscious or intentional process. This view resonates strongly with Psychology's best-known theory of denial – that denial is an unconscious defence mechanism that allows people to cope with anxiety, guilt or other disturbing emotions by simply 'blocking off' this information and preventing it from reaching the conscious mind (Cohen 2001: 5).

Denial can also vary in terms of what is being denied and how (*content*). According to Cohen this can be done in three different ways. The first is known as *literal denial*. It is the most simple and basic form of denial as it entails the blatant and literal denial of an event to suggest that 'it did not happen' (Cohen 2001: 7). However, denial needs not be the complete disavowal of an action or event. Cohen's other two distinctions are more subtle. Denial can also be a contestation of the conventional interpretation of an event. In this case the basic facts are admitted, but actors claim that what happened is 'not what you think it is, not what it looks like, not what you call it' (Cohen 2001: 7). This is known as *interpretive denial*. Finally, actors could both admit the basic facts and accept the conventional interpretation. However, the significance or implications of the event are then reformulated and rationalised in a manner that paves the way for 'justified' inaction through absolving the agents of any further responsibility. This is known as *implicatory denial* as essentially the implications of an event are debated. As the following chapters will show, South African government action shows elements of all of these approaches.

In the third category Cohen (2001: 10) differentiates amongst the various levels of *organisation* that are able to commit denial. On the simplest level there is individual, personal denial. This involves the individual psyche and therefore has close ties to the fields of Psychology and Psychoanalysis. The second organisational level considers official bodies – specifically governments. This form of denial is 'public, collective and highly organised' and is usually a means for a government to cover up or euphemise certain issues (Cohen 2001: 10). Official denial is of central concern to this study. Cohen's final distinction deals with the widest level of organisation – society. In this case, entire communities choose to maintain a lie. This collective effort is known as 'cultural denial' (Cohen 2001: 11).

The fourth facet of denial considers *time*. Denial can either be historical or contemporary. Memory, forgetting and repression are central to historical denial (Cohen 2001: 12). Whether they are victims, perpetrators or observers, individuals, officials or societies may resort to denial as a means of 'forgetting' the atrocities they have experienced, inflicted or witnessed. However, it is contemporary denial (the contestation of current events) that is most relevant in this book.

People, organisations or societies experience denial differently, depending on how they are implicated. To illustrate this, Cohen has mapped the agents of denial on what he calls an 'atrocity triangle'. The first corner is occupied by the victims who suffer a wrongdoing and then choose to deny this experience. This can also happen on the cultural or societal level (Cohen 2001: 14). In the second corner of the triangle is the perpetrator. Here those agents who have committed an unacceptable act find a way to deny it (in keeping with Cohen's typology, this can be either literal, interpretive or implicatory). The last corner of the 'atrocity triangle' is occupied by bystanders. Cohen (2001: 15) distinguishes amongst immediate bystanders, external bystanders and bystander states. In the case of the South African epidemic, government could be considered to at times have occupied all three corners of the triangle – victim, bystander and perpetrator (this is recalled again later in the discussion).

Finally, there is a distinction between *space and place*. According to Cohen (2001: 19) whether the act of denial is committed within the actor's own space and place or someone else's has a definite impact on the actors in terms of their own identity and political role (Cohen 2001: 19). In the South African case the space and place is the suspected denialist's own. Table 3.1 illustrates how South African government denial is positioned within these six determinants of denial.

Table 3.1 The elementary forms of denial

Psychological Status	Content	Organisation	Time	Agent	Space
Unconscious	Literal denial	Personal	Historical	Victim	Own
Conscious	Interpretive denial	Official	Contemporary	Bystander	Elsewhere
	Implicatory denial	Cultural		Perpetrator	

Source: Cohen (2001).

It is important to note that one common thread binds all such forms of denial – the supposition that there must be an ultimate truth (which the subject denying the fact must be aware of on some level) against which this denial can be measured. Without this underlying truth, it cannot technically be termed 'denial' (Cohen 2001: 6). In the case of the South African epidemic, as the preceding discussion has shown, evidence of the reality of HIV and AIDS abounds.

Cohen has built his typology of official denial around these elementary forms of denial to construct a repertoire of the various kinds of denial a government may resort to. Using Cohen's assessment of official denial it is possible to determine not only the extent to which denial may have resulted in official lethargy and inadequate response, but also to speculate on underlying political causes for this denial. When applied to a historical overview of South African government action, Cohen's typology should highlight both the presence and frequency of official denial. This then gives way to further insight into the possible motives that may have underlined government denial of the epidemic.

A typology of official denial

Cohen's typology differentiates amongst three broad variants of official denial. The first is 'classic official denial' and deals with the elementary forms of content denial as outlined above: literal, interpretive and implicatory denial. The second variant investigates instances in which officials attack their attackers ('counter-offensive denial'). This is done, amongst others, through accusing the accuser of lying, citing errors, claiming the move was politically motivated or otherwise discrediting the critics. The third variant is the most nuanced approach as it entails government partially acknowledging the issue but then finding some way to avoid further responsibility or obligation to action (Cohen 2001: 101). This strategy is quite simply referred to as 'partial acknowledgement'. Table 3.2 summarises Cohen's typology of official denial.

This typology does present one challenge – it draws mostly from single incidences of violence or atrocity that are then in some way euphemised, covered up or otherwise denied by officials. Previous applications of this typology have

Table 3.2 Cohen's typology of official denial

Classic Official Denial			Counter-offensive Denial	Partial Acknowledgement
Literal Denial	Interpretive Denial	Implicatory Denial		

Source: Cohen (2001).

also been limited to single issues. Hegarty (2004) has used it to assess officials' reactions to Bloody Sunday and Zerouali (1999) applied it to the Algerian Massacres. Welch (2003) has offered a slightly broader application of the typology in his discussion of official denial of human rights violations during the global war on terror.

The South African case on the other hand stretches over more than 25 years and deals with four different governments and a whole range of HIV and AIDS-related issues. To accommodate this, instead of treating denial as a single occurrence, incidents most suggestive of official denial since 1982 are identified and then categorised into Cohen's typology in order to achieve a measure of the extent to which the allegations of official denial hold true. This is done in two parts – an initial historical, chronological overview of government response sets a timeline from which possible instances of denial are then extracted and discussed thematically in the latter section of this book.

At this point it is important to note that official denial is most frequently found in government rhetoric – the communication resulting from interaction between key figures within a government and the media, the government's critics and supporters, as well as the general public. Often such communications are labelled propaganda, disinformation, spin or cover-up (Cohen 2001: 4, 102). Official denial is therefore not commonly found in policy or other official documentation but rather in the PR material of a government, including speeches and media reports. Analysing government actions for denial would therefore entail assessing the rhetoric and communications of key policy actors, which in this case would include the Minister of Health, other officials within the Department of Health, as well as the President. So far the term 'government' has predominantly been used to refer to 'officials' or 'policy makers'. All three terms will continue to be used interchangeably when appropriate, as the rhetoric in question is sometimes issued by one policy maker or alternatively by government officials collectively.

Cohen (2001: 102) further points out that an entire discourse of denial often emerges from claims and counterclaims and resultant exchanges about a particular issue between officials and those levelling criticism at them. Given the frequency with which governments respond to issues through the media and other public channels, this discourse often seems common practice and therefore is more likely to be perceived as a matter of public relations and spin, rather than as explicit denial and lies. This makes official denial challenging to argue convincingly as it tends to come across as a normal turn of events for most governments.

Modern, democratic denial is therefore less a matter of official silence and secrecy and more one of calculated response devised to create a perception amongst its critics and the general public that there is no issue. This comes as most modern states have little choice but to appease influential international bodies like the UN and the IMF and international opinion in general (Cohen 2001: 103). At this level the South African official response has been vociferous. Cameron (2000: 13) describes it as a 'cacophony of task groups, workshops, committees, councils, policies, drafts, proposals, statements, and pledges'. He further notes that 'piteously little' has come of these. Against Cohen's discussion of propaganda and other means of 'appeasing' critics, this could be interpreted as being consistent with officials' tactic of generating discourse that creates deceptions of good intention but ultimately falls short of action.

Conclusion

The long-wave nature of HIV and AIDS makes it virtually impossible to single out one particular government and hold it solely accountable for the severity and scale of the South African epidemic. Instead it is most likely to be the result of continued inaction and wilful neglect by all South African governments since 1982. Whilst the two Mbeki governments' foot dragging on treatment rollout in particular renders it morally questionable (some would say even genocidal), the truth is that by the time Mbeki came to power and AIDS became a popular topic much of the damage had already been done. It follows that long before ARVs were developed and prior to Mbeki and his governments' notorious handling of the epidemic South African officials responded to AIDS with insufficient urgency.

Should permutations of official AIDS denial be at least partially to blame for such inaction, such denial is likely to have been an equally long-standing affair and by no means limited to Mbeki. In this chapter the case was made for allegations of government denial to be extended beyond Mbeki and his governments. On this basis a denial hypothesis takes shape that suggests a possibility of government denial from the time when the first AIDS deaths were reported in South Africa until the end of the second Mbeki administration in September 2008. As this chapter has shown, the form of denial in question here refers not only to AIDS denialism as the contestation of mainstream AIDS science, but instead refers to a much broader form of denial in which any truth (not just scientific fact) is contested. Investigating these allegations of denial presents a number of challenges. Following a thorough review of existing research, Cohen's typology of official denial was identified as the most viable means of investigating South African government action, inaction and reaction to test the extent to which these allegations of government denial might hold true.

PART I
A History of the Official Response

Chapters 1, 2 and 3 have contextualised the main focus of this book, which will now be expounded in Parts I and II. In the course of the next three chapters (Part I) we tell the story of the South African AIDS epidemic as a chronological narrative. Chapter 4 describes the last two apartheid governments' responses to AIDS, from the very first indications in 1982 of what was to come to the tumultuous challenges of governing AIDS in the early 1990s, as the country was navigating a tenuous socio-political transition. Chapter 5 takes the story forward by focusing on the presidency of Nelson Mandela and Chapter 6 concludes our historical focus by recounting the incredible miscarriage of government that was Thabo Mbeki's response to the epidemic. When this historical discussion is cast against Cohen's typology of official denial, distinct possible instances of official denial become clear. Whilst these suspected incidents of government denial are briefly alluded to throughout the discussion in Part I, it is only in Part II that they are thoroughly dissected.

In Part II (Chapters 7–9) we change our analytical focus from a 'what' to a 'how and why' investigation into South African official AIDS denial specifically. We do this by taking the suspected instances of official denial that have been indentified in the historical narrative set out in Part I and categorising them into Cohen's typology of official denial.

The key difference between Parts I and II is that, whereas Part I sets out a chronological political history of the South African epidemic, Part II breaks that historical narrative into themes, for the sake of analytical clarity. This thematic overview reveals patterns and tendencies that point to possible underlying motives and drivers of government denial. It is therefore through application of Cohen's typology that a picture around the politics of AIDS denial begins to develop. This insight gained into how leadership might respond to long-wave events like HIV presents a valuable contribution to existing research around the epidemic.

Chapter 4
Past is Prologue: Apartheid Responses to AIDS

The terrorists are now coming to us with a weapon more terrible than Marxism: AIDS.

Pik Botha, apartheid Foreign Minister, 1987

Preparing the perfect storm

Apartheid South Africa provided a rich societal Petri dish within which HIV and AIDS could flourish. The epidemics of the past (for instance the Spanish flu after World War I) and the present (such as H1N1 in 2009) demonstrate that major epidemics do not crop up by chance. Instead they occur when circumstances offer a favourable breeding ground to pathogens. As is the case with individuals, a population's immunity to societal ills can be weakened by several co-factors, and the South Africa of 1982 (when the first AIDS deaths were recorded) was a society most vulnerable to HIV. This confirms Louis Pasteur's notion that '[t]he microbe is nothing; the terrain everything' (quoted in Serpa 2002: 43). The 'terrain', it is important to note, refers as much to biological factors as it does to non-biological ones, and hence the socio-political context of South Africa in the early 1980s is a significant determinant of the spread of the epidemic.

In 1982 South Africa was governed by a political party bent on racial separation and discrimination – the society was defined by an unequal distribution of resources, widespread poverty, the profligate duplication of civil services, international isolation[1] and regional military insurgencies, the absence of democracy and effective/good governance, domestic political instability, and gender inequality. At the time there was wide-spread ignorance about HIV and AIDS – given the fact that it was a newly identified pathogen, with very few victims, the reality was that politicians had very little incentive to immediately mobilise public resources to counter its impact. Furthermore, a complex set of cultural factors was playing a catalytic role in the environment within which AIDS was introduced. The social cohesion that is needed to combat HIV and AIDS was absent (and, some would say, continues to be absent to this day).

---

1 Whiteside (1991: 1) noted in the early 1990s that the majority of African countries had been able to call on the World Health Organisation (WHO) for assistance. Because of apartheid the WHO was unable to operate in South Africa in the 1980s and early 1990s.

Instead, as mentioned in Chapter 2, there were traditional social practices that fostered infection, a decaying social fabric, great female vulnerability, and an economic production system reliant on migratory labour (rural-urban, but regionally as well). All these factors created an environment of risk for the people of South Africa, and this risk was compounded by the fact that although AIDS was first recognised as a syndrome in 1981 and HIV as its cause in 1984, a systematic national and international response to the epidemic only started to take shape in 1986–87.[2] According to Dorrington and Johnson (2002: 14) this environment of risk was of such a magnitude that 'on any scale of high-risk situations South Africa in the 1980s ranked near the top'.

Initial responses

In the first few years after the first reported cases of AIDS in South Africa, the medical community founded a number of state-backed institutions and other formal bodies in order to formulate and implement some initial AIDS interventions. These interventions and institutions had a narrow focus on the virology of the HI virus, for the most part ignoring the social aspects of the epidemic (Moodie 1988: 58). Although the apartheid government's National Department of Health established a small AIDS Advisory Group (AAG) in 1985,[3] the most prominent institutional initiative was the establishment of the Medical Research Council's (MRC) AIDS Virus Research Unit (AVRU) in January 1987 – a full five years after the first reported AIDS fatality in South Africa. The mandate of the AVRU was to provide a centre for expertise for mostly biomedical studies on the HI virus, but even so the Unit did not envisage long-term research programmes, since 'the field of AIDS research [was] changing so rapidly that it [was] difficult to pinpoint long-term goals' (Editorial 1987: 15).

In the context of increasing criticism from civil society about the government's inaction about AIDS (even once F.W. De Klerk had assumed power in 1989)[4] the MRC formally launched its National AIDS Research Programme (NARP) in January 1992 – a full ten years after the first reported AIDS deaths in South Africa.

2 Fransen (1998: 6) notes that the WHO's Global Programme on AIDS (GPA) (the predecessor of UNAIDS) was established in 1986. Bilateral HIV prevention programmes in developing countries (from which apartheid South Africa was excluded), launched by the USA and the European Community (EC), were started in 1987.

3 Neither gays nor blacks were represented on SA's official AIDS Advisory Committee (Raphaely 1989: 15).

4 Holmshaw (1992: 149–50) stated that '[d]espite the two years' leeway afforded them by their isolation at the southern-most part of the continent,...[the government] is insisting on business as usual. The health planners at the Health Ministry have shown extreme reluctance to implement some of the feasible interventions as recommended by [the World Health Organisation]. They have also recently downgraded AIDS prevention efforts and put a stop to a comprehensive, innovative and promising communication and education campaign'.

The NARP was one of six national research programmes in the organisation and it is important to note for the first time provided for some analysis of the socio-political context of South African AIDS. Research projects undertaken by the NARP included seroprevalance studies, demographic projection studies, economic impact assessments, research into education and prevention efforts, and clinical care and counselling research (Steinberg 1993: 3).

In addition to the mainly biomedical research focus of the MRC's AVRU and then later on the NARP, two more structures were launched under the aegis of the medical community to combat HIV and AIDS. In the first instance, the South African Institute for Medical Research (SAIMR) established an AIDS Centre in January 1988. The main aim of the Centre was to promote AIDS education by presenting a series of one-day courses targeting different groups (Sherr et al. 1989). (However, as noted the central tenets of this information strategy were flawed).

Secondly, after 1987 it became increasingly obvious that a shift towards a more widespread epidemic was inevitable – more became known about the epidemiology and transmission vectors of the virus (Van Ammers 1990: 39). The government's Department of National Health and Population Development (NDHPD), focusing on the 'need for information' (McKerrow 2003: 2) and channelling resources through the SAIMR, created a number of AIDS Training and Information Centres (ATICS) in the cities and larger towns in the country.

South Africa's medical community in the 1980s suffered from divisive and inappropriate normative as well as legal frameworks, with the government providing precious little by way of developing a more appropriate and enabling biomedical response model. The epidemiological modelling that came into existence in later years provided too little information, too late, and the institutional structures that were set up came late in the day and were based on erroneous assumptions that disregarded or downplayed the socio-political environment within which the medical community had to operate. For the most part the government left this community to its own devices, undermining rather than enabling this critically important agent for an effective public sector response. Instead, the apartheid government attempted to criminalise and legislate AIDS away.

As we will later argue in greater detail in Part II, government's initial responses to the epidemic resonate with a number of variants of official denial as set out in Cohen's typology. The ineffectiveness of early reactive measures like setting up institutions to address HIV and AIDS, speak to elements of partial acknowledgement as a means to appease critics by appearing to take cognisance of the problem. However, as these promises do not translate into the necessary and required action, the sincerity of government's intentions is then brought into question. Given the relative lack of knowledge of the epidemic at the time, it is possible that government's lacklustre reaction was simply a result of their ignorance of the epidemic's devastating potential. However, the morally contested ethos that prevailed amongst government during the apartheid era underwrote many of these earlier reactions. And that AIDS at that time appeared to be limited to already disregarded and deplorable groups (homosexuals, commercial sex workers, intravenous drug users and later black people), hints towards slightly more questionable motives. Whilst government reaction at that time cannot be considered denial in the pure Freudian sense of disavowal, their construction of narratives around carrier groups does echo elements of Cohen's construction of official denial. This has been particularly apparent in government's early attempts at legislating against the issue.

In the absence of a strategy, legislate

The apartheid government's strategy regarding AIDS seemed to reflect an unwillingness or inability to deal with the socio-political structures underlying the unfolding epidemic, leaving it to other sections of South African society to muddle through on their own. In doing so, a policy of *inaction* rather than proactive planning and intervention seemed to be the government's approach. In the absence of an overall government strategy with regards to AIDS it became incumbent upon the biomedical community as well as sections of the private sector to draft their own context-specific and rather *ad hoc* policies. The private sector battled with conditions of employment in particular, struggling to come to grips with the implications of AIDS in the workplace.

Apartheid laws had criminalised certain forms of sexual relations that acted as a vector for the spread of HIV: homosexual relations, commercial sex work, as well as relations across racial divisions. In criminalising these aspects of South African sexual life, the apartheid government had their scapegoats, as well as an excuse for inaction: in the normative environment at the time, these kinds of activities (including intravenous drug use) were deemed as unnatural or morally reprehensible and thus the government's response to the deeper structural causes of the spread of the AIDS epidemic was to stigmatise, isolate and legislate against these forms of sexual relations. This was policy making by inaction rather than by the drafting of a proactive HIV and AIDS-specific set of programmes.

The white National Party (NP) government defined the AIDS problem in moralistic and racist terms: the HIV-positive individual was – due to their own immoral behaviour – responsible for their own infection. As such, that individual posed a danger to the rest of the 'normal' or 'innocent' society. The definition of the AIDS issue as a problem to which blame could be apportioned thus found application in legislation based on an attempt to censure and even criminalise those in which the AIDS issue became personalised. In the absence of a human rights charter in the normative and highly politicised[5] AIDS policy environment it comes

5 The personalisation of AIDS soon became a political tool. When four ANC members, imprisoned for alleged terrorism, were diagnosed as HIV-positive in the mid-to-late 1980s, the then South African Minister of Foreign Affairs, Pik Botha, declared that '…[t]he terrorists are now coming to us with a weapon more terrible than Marxism: AIDS' (quoted in Kirby 1993: 13).

as no surprise that the apartheid government's lack of an encompassing AIDS policy resulted in an attempt to simply legislate the issue into oblivion. According to Kirby (1993: 1), panic, alarm, banishment, cruelty, public stigmatisation and (significantly) *law* are 'the melancholy companions of disease and epidemics', and in South Africa it was no different – the AIDS-specific legislation enacted by the apartheid government actually exacerbated the AIDS problem, rather than ameliorating it. Such laws 'impede an effective response to the epidemic. They block the educational messages that are essential to behaviour modification and containment of the spread [...] One of the real dangers of AIDS is that it will produce a new virus of HIL – Highly Inefficient Laws' (Kirby 1993: 2, 3).

The first AIDS-specific piece of legislation that the apartheid government enacted was the *Human Tissue Act* (65 of 1983) that the government amended in 1990. In accordance with this legislation, particular groups of people were excluded as blood donors – gay men in particular (Van Wyk 1992b). The standard test for HIV only became available in 1985, so the aim of the legislation was to draw attention to those individuals who were thought to be of risky donors, and by implication to protect the rest of the population against their unsafe blood. As was the case with the later *Immorality Amendment Act* (2 of 1988), the effect of this legislation was that isolated and stigmatised groups were actually driven deeper underground, in fact not declaring their sexual orientation or risky sexual partnering for fear of legal prosecution. According to Burchell (1990: 195):

> [l]egislation aimed at curbing the spread of AIDS...can be categorized as imposing either direct or indirect control to prevent the communication of HIV to new victims. Indirect action might take the form of criminalizing aspects of homosexuality, prostitution, drug-taking and drug-peddling. It is surely not entirely coincidental that the *Immorality Amendment Act* 2 of 1988, although ostensibly designed to remove discrimination in the field of sexual offences, in fact expands the field of criminality in the area of prostitution and the activities of escort agencies at a time when the fear of the spread of AIDS has begun to take hold in South Africa.

The most significant AIDS-specific legislation of the apartheid government was announced on 30 October 1987 (Strauss 1988: 14).[6] On that day the Minister of National Health and Population Development published amendments to the *Public Health Act* (63 of 1977) that gave special powers to medical officers of health with regards to HIV-positive individuals. Until then, AIDS was not a notifiable disease, but under the new regulations a medical officer that suspected someone to be the carrier of a communicable disease could instruct that person to subject him/herself to a medical examination. The regulations further provided that if a person in the opinion of a medical officer was – or could be – suffering from any communicable disease mentioned in the regulations (one of which was AIDS), that person

6 Cameron (1991b: 195) lamented as late as 1991 that aside from these two pieces of legislation, 'Parliament itself has not addressed the issue...'.

was to subject themselves to a medical examination and treatment as could be subsequently prescribed. If a person was found to be a carrier of HIV, the Minister was also afforded the power to place that person in quarantine – ominously, 'until he is free of infection' (Cameron 1991b: 195).

These regulations did not render AIDS a fully notifiable medical condition. If it had, all persons who might have had reason to believe that a person had died from it would have had to report this fact to the local authority. A medical practitioner who treated a person suffering from a notifiable medical condition had to submit weekly reports on the patient to the regional director of health. However, these conditions were not prescribed for AIDS. HIV and AIDS were merely added to a list of 'communicable diseases' provided for in the *Public Health Act*. The effect was to render AIDS notifiable to a limited extent and to bring into play the possibility of compulsory hospitalisation or isolation of persons suspected of having contracted the syndrome (Burchell 1990: 196).

Interestingly, however, the amendments to the *Health Act* also meant that local authorities had the power to shut public service agencies and even schools could be closed to an HIV-positive individual – even a pupil.[7] The amendments obligated school principals to notify medical officers of the presence of an HIV-positive pupil or staff member – such notification had to take place even if school principals only suspected an individual of being HIV-positive (Beckmann and Prinsloo 1993: 52; Southern African Practice Management 1988: 5).

Another important regulation published on the same day (30 October 1987) by the Minister of Home Affairs related to diseases that would render foreigners who find themselves on South African soil 'prohibited persons' for the purposes of the *Admission of Persons to the Republic Regulation Act*. One of the conditions listed in the regulation was AIDS (or infection with HIV). The Act empowered immigration officers to require *inter alia* persons who in their opinion are not entitled to be in the Republic to submit to a medical examination where there was a suspicion that the person concerned was afflicted with a listed disease. The fact that a foreigner would become a 'prohibited person' did not mean that they would necessarily be required to leave the country, or be deported. The Act did, however, vest the Minister with wide powers of deporting non-citizens if it was deemed in the public interest.

Civil rights activists immediately stated their opposition to these two pieces of legislation, warning that the implications of the legislation – in particular its slant towards making AIDS a notifiable disease – enforced the environment of apportioning blame. This would, in their opinion, only serve to drive the disease even deeper underground, enforcing stigmatisation and discrimination (Cameron 1991b: 197). Once the ANC and other liberation organisations were unbanned on 2 February 1990 these civil rights activists indicated that this legislation (which

---

7 The provisions of the *Education Affairs Act* (70 of 1988) supported this legislation, stating that, although it is compulsory for all children between seven and 16 years of age to attend school, a child could be exempted from compulsory school attendance as a result of continuous ill-health (due to factors including HIV and AIDS) (Oosthuizen 1994: 253).

provided immigration officials with the right to deny individuals even suspected of being HIV-positive access to the country, or to deport non-nationals to other countries) could be used against returning political exiles. In short, the legislation could be used to politicise and racialise the issue of AIDS even more.

Significantly, opposition to these measures was such that they became almost instantly unenforceable. Shortly after the enactment of the new measures in the *Public Health Act* and the *Admission of Persons to the Republic Regulation Act*, the government announced plans to repatriate 1,000 Malawian miners who had tested HIV-positive and to have all work applicants from Malawi, Zimbabwe, Zambia, Zaire and Burundi tested for the virus.[8] However, the deportation plans were thwarted by doctors who reportedly refused to disclose the names of infected miners to the government on the strength of the duty of doctor-patient confidentiality (Cameron and Swanson 1992: 498).

However, the government's plans to implement pre-employment testing of work applicants from Central Africa did go forward. In fact, in 1986 and 1987, even before AIDS and HIV were added to the scheduled conditions, all persons seeking employment in South African mines who originated from what the Minister of National Health and Population Development termed 'high risk areas' were tested before being allowed to work in South African mines. However, once the change in the AIDS policy environment moved towards a more human rights-centred approach, the Chamber of Mines altered their policy and entered into negotiations with the National Union of Mineworkers (NUM) on this issue (Cameron and Swanson 1992: 499).

As political changes in South Africa accelerated after 2 February 1990, the anachronistic and untenable nature of these pieces of legislation became increasingly apparent. In April 1991, therefore, the apartheid government's AIDS Unit published a policy document pragmatically rejecting the use of coercive legislation in the fight against AIDS – in effect rejecting both pieces of the 30 October 1987 legislation. In June 1991 the government-appointed AIDS Advisory Committee recommended that legislation stigmatising AIDS and HIV be repealed. As a result, in October 1991, AIDS and HIV were dropped from the immigration regulations, and indications were that AIDS may also be removed from the communicability regulations. At that time Cameron (1993: 23) noted that:

> [t]hese changes are important. They signal that the government has accepted that statutory coercion has no useful part to play in fighting the spread of HIV. This is a vital lesson; once South Africans had the benefit of learning through the bitter history of the *Immorality Act* 23 of 1957, which showed that punitive and stigmatizing laws cannot control the way people behave: they cause only misery and devastation while bringing the law and its enforcers into disrepute.

8 When the testing indicated a high incidence of HIV amongst workers from Malawi, the government of Malawi refused the further testing of their nationals migrating to South Africa for work. This is why the supply of Malawian workers dried up very early.

Elsewhere, Cameron and Swanson (1992: 499) noted that:

> [t]he change in the law also reveals an important general shift in the government's approach to the growing AIDS epidemic. By removing the prohibition on immigrants with HIV or AIDS, the government has implicitly acknowledged that South Africa cannot insulate itself from the crisis by establishing a 'cordon sanitaire' around the country.

In short, the government had moved from a position of wanting to pass legislation that criminalised those deemed responsible for spreading HIV and AIDS, to a position that appeared to embrace those individuals' human rights. There was clearly an implicit shift in the definition of the AIDS problem. This shift will be discussed in greater detail below. But first, the impact and changes in South African Criminal and Case Law on the broader legal environment will be evaluated.

As is the case in contemporary South Africa, during apartheid it was illegal for commercial sex workers to practice their trade in the open, and hence it was very difficult to target this group for AIDS intervention programmes. Also criminalised during apartheid were homosexual relationships as well as sexual relations between people of different races. In doing so the government's response to AIDS was to target specific sectors of South African society and blame them for the spread of the epidemic. The enemy was not a virus; the enemy was the individual who – through their own morally unacceptable actions – posed a threat to the rest of society. Such a policy of blame would naturally find application in the use of Criminal Law: by criminalising the conduits of the virus, government could be seen to act in the interests of the greater constituency that they represented – white heterosexuals. It is likely that this initial apportioning of the blame to groups on the fringes of society was motivated, at least to an extent, by government's unwillingness to acknowledge the real causes and potential dangers of HIV and AIDS. However, relying on legislation to contain the HI virus meant that government facilitated and sanctioned the construction a number of controversial (and scientifically incorrect) messages around HIV and AIDS. Legislating against the issue suggested, for one, that AIDS did not kill morally upstanding citizens but only homosexuals, drug users, prostitutes and/or black people. By deduction, law-abiding citizens were thus entirely insulated from infection. Apart from irrevocably stigmatising the disease as a consequence of morally reprehensible activity and deeply racialising the epidemic, these messages speak to Cohen's construction of literal and implicatory official denial. We explore this in more detail in Chapter 8. It is quite telling that, by the time in the late 1980s when it started to become apparent that the AIDS epidemic would be a chiefly heterosexual phenomenon, government's emphasis on using Criminal Law to ostensibly combat the epidemic also died down.

Criminal Law was thus used by the NP government as a way to force individuals to alter their sexual behaviour (De Jager 1991: 214). In doing so South African Criminal Law was used to perpetuate the framing of the AIDS epidemic in 'us versus them' terms: the Criminal Law environment at the time made all South

Africans either vectors of victims of the disease – and if you were a vector, you could be punished for it. De Jager (1991: 216–17) cites two reasons in particular to explain why this application of Criminal Law did not succeed.

In the first place, the coercive nature of what Criminal Law implied had the effect of exculpating individuals who might deem themselves as 'victims' rather than 'vectors'. In targeting sexual and other outsiders as criminals, the use of Criminal Law made it possible for the rest of society to not take responsibility for their own sexual acts. Secondly, the application of Criminal Law as a tacit policy tool to cope with AIDS was based on the assumption that individuals who spread the disease – the ones being criminalised – would remain in their designated (outlawed) groups, and that criminalisation would be enough to isolate the virus to homosexuals, sex workers, drug users and non-South African blacks. The government assumed that, in targeting these groups by criminalising them, they could protect the rest of society from viral transmission. This was clearly not the case, since by the late 1980s the general heterosexual nature of the epidemic started to become apparent.

In addition to the government's use of Criminal Law, the legal precedents of South African Case Law in the late 1980s and early 1990s provide some insight into how the government came to shape its evolving response set to AIDS. In the absence of a comprehensive government policy to deal with the legal aspects of HIV and AIDS, civil law cases were important determinants of the legal culture of South Africa after the democratisation of the country in April 1994. Between 1982 and 1994 there were two cases in particular that would shape the legal and policy environment in the years to come.

In the first of these – the McGeary case of 1991[9] – a civil court case resulted after a medical doctor disclosed a patient's HIV status to two colleagues whilst playing golf. The plaintiff's position was that his moral right to privacy had been violated by what he deemed his doctor's unprofessional action. In 1993 the South African Court of Appeal emphasised and supported the importance of the South African Medical and Dental Council's (SAMDC) 1989 guidelines on HIV and AIDS, which stated that it was the doctor's duty to protect a patient's right to confidentiality if specifically asked to do so (which was the case here).

The case was important in that it legally bound any future South African policy making and legislation to the principle of patient confidentiality, rendered the SAMDC guidelines legally enforceable, and considered the HIV-positive patient's right to privacy as more pressing that the actual risks associated with occupational HIV transmission.[10] The message to South African public policy makers was that the tide was turning: away from using the law as a tool to further stigmatise

---

9 For greater detail on the evolution of this case, see the *Journal of Contemporary Roman-Dutch Law* (1992), *Southern African Practice Management* (1992), the *Annual Survey of South African Law* (1993) and Sarkin (1993).

10 The McGeary decision also provided greater clarity in light of an earlier decision, in 1989, in which the court ruled that the confidential relationship between doctor and

and criminalise the HIV-positive individual, towards respecting the rights of that individual, and making policy adjustment in accordance with that implication.

The Hansen case of 1992 is the second civil case that had important implications for AIDS policy making in South Africa. In this case, the plaintiff took the administration of a hospital to court because the latter refused to provide him with further free medication for which he had previously qualified, whilst continuing the free provision of the medication to HIV negative patients. The hospital's decision to do so was based on pecuniary considerations, stating that the right of a patient to free medication became effectively curtailed if that patient were HIV-positive, because the medication would cost the state too much money, especially in view of the fact that the patient would die in the long run. In its decision, the court discarded this argument, stating that all patients should be treated equally – regardless of their HIV status.

The implication of the court's decision was that the government would be forced to cease discriminating against HIV-positive individuals, and adjust legislation accordingly to provide such individuals with life-saving drugs. More importantly, however, was the implication that the government and all South Africans needed to take personal but also communal responsibility for AIDS. As Chetty (1993: 76) stated just after the decision was publicised, '[i]t should become the moral and social obligation of all citizens to take active measures in making war against AIDS, and not against people with AIDS'. As with the McGeary decision, the Hansen case forced the South African legal context and government away from the spirit of blame and stigmatisation to combating the disease as a societal phenomenon that should be tackled by expanding rather than contracting individuals' human rights.

The move to a human rights culture

Taken as a whole, the evolution of private sector and legal measures to combat AIDS discussed above indicates the emergence of an interesting trend by the early 1990s, which informed the public policy environment: despite the government's efforts to demonise HIV-positive individuals in the workplace and legislate against them in South African society as a whole, the occupational and legal elites refused to ideologically embrace and implement governmental prescriptions. Human resources managers, insurance portfolio managers and the courts discarded the implications of government's tacit AIDS policy, and opted instead to rephrase their own sectoral response to AIDS in a human rights discourse. At the core of this disassociation was a dissonance with government's racist-moralist position on AIDS, namely that the personalised vectors of the epidemic should be held morally responsible for endangering the rest of society.

---

patient was subject to legal limitations. For information on that case, see *Davis v Additional Magistrate, Johannesburg 1989 (4) SA 299 (W) at 303E-I.*

In doing so, these elites in the implementation of what tacit governmental AIDS policies there were refused to be a party to those policies. The very fact that some influential sectors of South African society acted counter to the prescriptions of the government – discarding their moralistic stance in the process – demonstrates the power of a new mindset based on individual human rights. There was a clear contrast between the way in which the government perceived the reality of AIDS (zero-sum, namely the rights of the many versus the rights of the few), and the way in which others came to view the epidemic (namely that the virus is the problem, rather than the individuals spreading it). Eventually even the AIDS managers within the government (namely, the AIDS Advisory Committee) in June 1991 also arrived at this changed position, which led to the eventual repeal of discriminatory AIDS legislation four months later. After October 1991, it was clear that AIDS would be seen as less of a health issue, and as more of a developmental, social justice and human rights issue.[11]

Reviewing the AIDS legal context of the late 1980s, Cameron (1993: 22) warned that – should the October 1987 legislation have been allowed to continue – discrimination against people with AIDS could well have replaced racism as the major focus of exclusionary conduct in South Africa. In Cameron's analysis the 1987 legislation exemplified the three forms of discrimination that there could have been with regards to people living with AIDS:

- The enactment by the state of repressive laws aimed at inhibiting civil liberties or civic status of persons with AIDS or HIV.
- The violation by health-care workers, employers and others of HIV-positive individual's first generation rights – the rights to dignity, privacy and autonomy; and
- Denying persons with AIDS or HIV access to a fair share of national resources and wealth, in both the public and the private sectors (second generation rights).

The repeal of the October 1987 legislation as well as the civil courts' decisions in the early 1990s against similar legislation was therefore a major victory for human rights activists, since:

> [i]t [was] in these areas that the human rights battle around AIDS and HIV over the next 15 years in South Africa [would] lie. It [would] not be primarily about 'first generation' rights. It [would] be the struggle for people with AIDS and HIV to get a fair and rational share of our nation's resources (Cameron 1993: 26).

11 For an overview of this reperception or redefinition of AIDS as a human rights issue rather than as a mere health problem, see FitzSimons (1990/91), Ulin (1992), Cameron and Swanson (1992), Leech (1993), Leech (1994), Kirby (1993b), Cameron (1993b), Heydt (1993), Strode (1994) and Kirby (1993).

Perhaps it comes as no surprise that this altered conception of the AIDS *problematique* happened at the time that it did: shortly after the tumultuous political changes announced by the President F.W. De Klerk in February 1990. The trade unions in particular found their voice, and it is significant that it was at its recent 1989 congress that the Congress of South African Trade Unions (COSATU) had made explicit their demands for a more holistic, human rights-centred approach to HIV and AIDS, followed shortly thereafter by the Transport and General Workers' Union's similar 1990 resolution on AIDS (COSATU 1991). The white government could no longer afford to merely suppress or discard its new constitutional negotiation partners' views on public policy issues, and it became clear that the normative AIDS environment was moving swiftly away from the Botha government's actions to criminalise the disease and stigmatise those held responsible for its dissemination.

The radically changed political context was underscored by the real need to change South African society's perception of previously rejected sexual behaviour. For instance, there were calls for the moral approval and decriminalisation of homosexuality, with Viljoen (1993: 114) enjoining public policy makers to 'replace punishment with empathy'. Moreover, AIDS activists and members of the medical elite within government agencies started to put pressure on the government to decriminalise commercial sex work, and to empower women by enacting greater gender equity (Sher 1990: 3). These notions where supported by a change within the South African medical community: less of an emphasis was placed on first world medicine, with greater emphasis on the notion of 'well-being', primary health care and the need for greater integration amongst the various schools of thought regarding individuals' rights to health – not only as a medical issue, but as a developmental issue (Yach 1992: 39).

The redefinition of AIDS as a human rights issue reached its civil society zenith on 12 November 1991, when the South African AIDS Consortium (an organisation representing the width and breadth of the AIDS civil society community) adopted its 'Charter of Rights on AIDS and HIV' (AIDS Consortium 1993). The Charter stressed the need to protect individuals' first and second generation rights in the context of AIDS, with specific reference to liberty, autonomy, confidentiality and privacy.

After February 1990 and increasingly after the repeal of discriminatory AIDS legislation in October 1991, it became clear that the AIDS problem had been redefined; the AIDS public policy environment had changed, ostensibly irrevocably.

The political governance of AIDS: 1982–94

Upon reviewing the NP government's actions and inactions on AIDS in the years following the first recorded AIDS mortality in South Africa in 1982, three loosely defined phases of AIDS governance for the era 1982–94 can be identified. Although it is difficult to provide meaningful, accurate timeframes to policy making, it is nonetheless possible to discern a first phase that stretched from 1982 until about 1988 – this era is notable for government inaction on AIDS. In fact, Van der Vliet (2004: 50) refers to these years as the 'silent' HIV phase.

The second phase of the public response to AIDS was from around 1989 to 1992, and is notable for the government's AIDS policy evolution to a more human rights-centred approach (yet still excluding the majority of public stakeholders in the broader policy environment). The third phase commenced with the establishment of the broadly inclusive National AIDS Co-ordinating Committee of South Africa (NACOSA) in 1992, and the development of the country's first truly encompassing, broadly inclusive AIDS strategy, culminating in the democratically elected ANC government adopting the National AIDS Plan (NAP) shortly after assuming office in 1994.

The 'silent' HIV phase: 1982–88

In the first few years after AIDS appeared on the South African political landscape the battle against the epidemic struggled – and, indeed, failed – to make it onto the public agenda. No comprehensive AIDS strategies or public policies were drafted. There are a number of reasons for this, but the most significant of these was that AIDS did not at first appear to be a truly dramatic threat to South African society.[12] At first there was no way of isolating and measuring the prevalence of the disease amongst South Africans, and very little was known about its possible impact. Also, the virus appeared to have the greatest impact amongst isolated fringes of South African society, affecting mainly homosexuals, commercial sex workers and intravenous drug users – sections of society who had already been legislated against; indeed, criminalised. There was no great pressure on the government to ease the burden that AIDS placed on these groups; rather, government acted to protect the rest of 'normal' South African society against these 'enemies within'.

As a consequence, it was easier to equate the real AIDS threat to South Africa with these peripheral groups. The problem on the public agenda was not to combat a virus that threatened the whole country; rather, the threat was the immoral behaviour of fringe groups who had brought this ill-defined plight upon themselves in the first place. The government's actions were, therefore, fairly predictable: a handful of pieces of legislation was drafted to restrict the behaviour of those individuals who were deemed to threaten the rest of society – foreign mine workers would be tested, immigrants would be scanned, homosexuals were excluded as blood donors, and immigration officials were given special powers to deport HIV-positive migrants. Rather than giving thought to extending the privileges and most basic human rights of blacks, gays, drug users and prostitutes,

---

12 According to Whiteside (1998: 89–91) this lack of threat perception was the result of the fact that, at first, AIDS appeared not be an immediate and credible threat to the majority of South Africans. There was no reliable source of data, and the epidemic appeared to be isolated amongst gays, sex workers and drug users.

the NP government acted to strengthen discriminatory legislation against these 'enemies'. It is quite likely that this reaction was underwritten by some form of official denial. The construction of these enemy groups meant the government created alternative truths around the epidemic. These included suggestions that HIV affected black citizens more than white ones and that by being a morally upstanding citizen one could avoid contracting the virus. When categorised into Cohen's typology, these statements suggest that some elements of denial may have been present in these early government responses.

In addition, the government in 1985 established the AIDS Advisory Group (AAG) to inform and drive its strategy on HIV and AIDS – a body comprised wholly of white men with leanings towards a narrow biomedical definition of the society-epidemiology interface. The resultant biomedical focus limited the drafting of AIDS policies that, in Klouda's (1994: 39) analysis, could go beyond 'being a mess': there was no recognition of the social services required to recognise, treat and support HIV-positive individuals, too few resources were allocated on the whole, and the biomedical focus never moved to address the primary health care initiatives that would be required to provide an appropriate response to the socio-epidemiological environment. This conception of the AIDS policy problem meant that the appropriate policies would never be implemented: '[t]he cosy compartments in which so many of us have placed the world have been shown to be irrelevant to reality' (Klouda 1994: 39). Hambridge (1990: 39) echoes this sentiment, stressing the fact that the 'medicalisation' of AIDS – viewing it as a health problem exclusively – blinded policy makers to the importance of social conditions that maximised the spread of the epidemic (for example urbanisation, urban poverty, hostel residences on the mines, political violence and gender imbalances).

Only towards the end of this era did the government establish a number of institutions to combat AIDS – and these remained exclusive and limited in number. Rather than addressing the structural causes for the rapid dissemination of AIDS in South Africa, these bodies were focused on medical solutions, reactively seeking to prevent the spread of the epidemic by way of ill-conceived and societally inappropriate information campaigns.[13] These campaigns were notable for their lack of sensitivity: many campaigns were only conducted in Afrikaans and English, were viewed by black South Africans as racist, and served to demonise HIV-positive individuals rather than being instructive on the main cause of AIDS: the HI virus itself (Van der Vliet 2004b: 49).

Limited as they were, it is significant that improvements only occurred once it became apparent in 1988 that AIDS had made the jump from the homo- to the heterosexual section of society: the 'gay plague' had become the 'black death' – an untimely addition to the greater NP pathology of a 'swart gevaar' [black danger]. This politicised the South African AIDS epidemic: the stigmatisation

13 For greater detail regarding criticism of the government's campaign, see Setiloane (1991: 5–7).

accompanying the virus and institutionalised in legislation was now exported to the broader context of South Africa's race politics – the NP government warned against ANC cadres importing the virus into the country, and the ANC blamed the NP government and Western powers for cooking up the virus in their laboratories to act as a weapon against blacks (Van der Vliet 2004a: 50).[14] Throw into this political cauldron the normative blame games played by leading South African churches at the time, and it becomes clear how the epidemic became so firmly and irretrievably politicised and racialised.

The country would pay the price for this for many years to come – an illegitimate government would henceforth find it increasingly difficult to secure the buy-in and ownership of their AIDS policies by the majority of South Africans,[15] AIDS remained erroneously defined as a personification amongst certain sections of society, and the narrow biomedical, health-specific policy response became the safest option of policy and decision makers. It is little wonder then that the NP government continuously fell short of the successful drafting of any comprehensive, circumspect and all-inclusive policy response to HIV and AIDS: the political environment made it near impossible to isolate and address the real drivers of the epidemic, the policy problem remained erroneously defined, and ineffectual, impotent policy responses inevitably followed suit.

Flux and reconceptualisation: 1989–92

The year 1989 was important in the political history of South Africa, as well as in the evolution of the country's governance of HIV and AIDS. By that time it became clear to the government that its policy of 'no explicit AIDS policy' was no longer tenable: the AIDS burden until then had been borne by individual households, the private sector and the biomedical community, but the government was now faced with an avalanche of calls from civil society, the business community and from within sectors of government itself to be more proactive in its approach to the emerging epidemic.

Also, the political landscape was changing: President P.W. Botha's stroke in early 1989 was the first step towards the F.W. De Klerk administration that

---

14 AIDS was, in fact, used by the NP government as an apartheid weapon: during the Truth and Reconciliation Commission (TRC) hearings in 1999 it was revealed that apartheid-era security officers strategically 'planted' HIV-positive operatives at two Johannesburg brothels with the explicit instruction to infect black sex workers (Whiteside and Sunter 2000: 65).

15 As anti-apartheid activist and medical doctor, Dr Ivan Toms, argued at the time, there was 'no possibility that the [National Party] government could, even it if had the inclination, run an effective campaign to limit the spread of HIV infection. It has no credibility or legitimacy whatsoever among blacks' (Van der Vliet 2004a: 52). Marais (2000: 6) echoes this sentiment, noting that '[i]n 1990–94…what was unavailable was the institutional and political stability…necessary to implement a coherent and co-ordinated response'.

formally assumed office in September of that year, as well as the unbanning of the liberation movements and the concomitant birth of the political transition period in February 1990. The normative policy environment now had to take greater note of the wishes and values of the government's negotiation partners (the ANC and their Mass Democratic Movement alliance partners), the South African legal system was no longer tolerant of the discriminatory legislation that had existed with regards to HIV-positive individuals in earlier years, and the McGeary as well as Hansen civil court cases indicated a powerful move towards and broadly supportive of the ANC and labour unions' insistence on the extension of basic human rights to the majority of South Africans – including people living with HIV and AIDS.[16]

As noted above, the government was forced to repeal the discriminatory legislation regarding AIDS that had been enacted in 1987, and the National Department of Health established a number of intragovernmental and other agencies to combat the epidemic. Also, it was clear that the NP government could no longer refuse the call to draft a comprehensive policy on AIDS[17] – putting an end to reactive, inappropriate, *ad hoc* and ill-conceived strategies that aimed at either apportioning blame, or at a biomedical 'solution' to the problem of AIDS. In the early 1990s, therefore, the NP government set out to draft a more appropriate policy on the epidemic (Ngwena and Pelser 2001: 2).

However, the fact that the government maintained its exclusion of the broader political players, civil society and AIDS activists; that nothing could change the fact that it was an illegitimate government to start off with; as well as that it was focusing primarily on constitutional negotiations with the ANC and the other liberation movements – all these factors meant that the AIDS policy environment remained difficult to navigate, with no comprehensive, inclusive and successful strategy on AIDS emerging. Despite this failure, it is important to note that the process of the redefinition of the AIDS policy problem did commence in the three years following on the changed political environment of 1989 – and the successful drafting of a truly democratised policy on AIDS would depend squarely on this redefinition.[18]

16 Both the ANC and the labour movement in South Africa held conferences on HIV and AIDS in the late 1980s and early 1990s (see AIDS Scan 1990, Draft Maputo Statement 1991, Labour Bulletin 1989). Just after being unbanned in 1990, the ANC also undertook to test its exile communities in Zambia and Tanzania for the HI virus before the majority of these cadres returned to South Africa (AIDS Analysis Africa 1991: 4).

17 According to Crewe (2000: 23) the absence of a comprehensive public policy on HIV and AIDS and the NP government strategy of haphazard and reactive measures aiming to merely provide biomedical information on how the virus is disseminated is one of the main features of South Africa's failure to combat the disease in the first decade of its presence in South African society.

18 Sadie and Van Aardt's (1992: 89–93) main points of criticism against the South African AIDS policy environment during this period was the fact that these were the years during which the politicisation of AIDS became the most entrenched, the fact that the NP government was seen as wholly illegitimate (thus rendering policy measures largely

The democratisation of AIDS governance: 1992–94

The redefinition of the AIDS policy problem as a human rights and development issue and its ensuing repositioning on the public agenda – with the greater need to include the key decision makers – led, in 1992, to a conference entitled 'South Africa united against AIDS' including members of the ruling NP government, key ANC officials, trade unionists, AIDS activists as well as members of the medical community. For the first time the main decision makers in the South African AIDS arena congregated and this development led to the establishment of a truly inclusive body – the National AIDS Co-ordinating Committee of South Africa (NACOSA). The latter would act as a kind of an 'AIDS caucus' where AIDS stakeholders could meet and develop a truly democratic response to the epidemic. The 1992 meeting that established NACOSA was described by AIDS policy analysts as 'an unusual show of national unity at a time of complex and sensitive political negotiations, well before an election date for a democratically elected government had been decided' (Nattrass 2004: 42).

By 1992 the newly instituted national antenatal HIV surveys made the extent of the reality of AIDS in South Africa clear to the reading public. The normative environment had shifted away from an exclusive conception of the AIDS policy problem, and now emphasised and embraced the need for a human rights-based approach to the epidemic. It was this confluence of a changed policy environment, the inclusion of the majority of important AIDS stakeholders and a sense of urgency that led to the drafting of South Africa's first comprehensive national strategy on HIV and AIDS: the National AIDS Plan (NAP – also known as 'the Plan') that was adopted within the first few months of the ANC assuming power in 1994.[19]

The successful drafting of the broadly popular NAP underscores the need for coherent political leadership in the establishment of an appropriate strategy to combat AIDS. According to Barnett and Whiteside (2002: 335) '[a] necessary... criterion for preventing spread of HIV or turning the epidemic round is political leadership...South Africa provides an example where absence of clear and decisive leadership damaged prevention activity'. In retrospect the truth of this statement is clear: for the first decade of AIDS in South Africa there was a deficit in the political will and leadership to appropriately combat the rapidly growing

impotent), the continued exclusion of the ANC and other major political groupings from the policy making environment, the ridiculously small budget that the government allocated for combating AIDS, as well as the insistence on an exclusive biomedical focus regarding the epidemic. Their criticism regarding the budget seems particularly accurate – and is easily verifiable: in 1987 R1 million was spent on AIDS prevention, in 1989 R5.4 million, and in 1992 only R23 million, of which about a third went to a single advertising agency. The 1993 budget was increased by only one per cent! (Whiteside 1993: 1).

19 As the NAP of 1994 was implemented under the Mandela government (1994–99), its main tenets will be reviewed and discussed as part of the evaluation of the AIDS governance specific to that era. (See the next chapter).

epidemic.[20] It was only once that political will came about and was translated into a reconceptualisation of the policy problem that an appropriate and widely praised strategy could be drafted. Significantly, two members of the core team within NACOSA that was responsible for the actual drafting of the NAP would go on to become consecutive Health Ministers in the new South African government: Drs Nkosazana Dlamini-Zuma and Manto Tshabalala-Msimang.

20 In 1991 Cameron (1991b: 194–5) noted that 'the law says little specifically about HIV infection and AIDS. Parliament itself has not addressed the issue…'. As late as 1994 Sadie, Van Aardt and Verwey (1994: 73, 76) noted that 'at present there is no legislation with regard to HIV and AIDS…it is generally agreed that the AIDS issue is of crucial importance and that large-scale action in the form of a comprehensive prevention strategy is essential'.

Chapter 5
The Mandela Government's Response to AIDS

> I wanted to win [the 1994 election] and I didn't talk about AIDS.
>
> Nelson Mandela

> In 199 ways he was our country's saviour. In the 200th way he was not.
>
> Edwin Cameron

After South Africa's first fully democratic elections on 27 and 28 April 1994 the country entered a honeymoon period: after months of political violence and nervous negotiations there was a remarkable absence of any violence during the actual election, the messianic Nelson Mandela was sworn in without incident as Head of State on 10 May 1994 and a new Government of National Unity (GNU) including former political foes was legitimately governing a truly democratic country. In short, the 'South African dream' had become a reality: four years of at times exceedingly tenuous political negotiations had paid off, and immediately the new political elite had to face the challenges of leadership.

Echoing the general sense of optimism that prevailed after Mandela's inauguration, Archbishop Desmond Tutu stated that '[o]nce we have got it right, South Africa will be the paradigm for the rest of the world' (quoted in Sparks 2003: 3). One of the reasons for the failure of the NAP might be exactly this spirit of hope. As Van der Vliet (2004b: 54) was to remark in retrospect:

> 1994 also was a time when the new government would prioritise positive programmes, such as housing, jobs, education and wider healthcare issues. AIDS warnings and the message of safer sex were not subjects congenial to those savouring the euphoria of freedom.

The new government inherited a polity in disarray: the NP government had created superfluous institutions and wasted money on replicating various state infrastructures in the so-called 'black homelands'. Economically, the country was institutionally isolated from external sources of liquidity, and close to insolvency. There was an urgent need to integrate the various governmental institutions and structures, get the economy growing, create jobs and foster greater socio-economic equality, finalise the constitution, and embark upon the challenges of nation-building.

Lurking above all of these immediate priorities was the reality of HIV and AIDS – but even this challenge did not seem insurmountable. After all, as described in the previous chapter, the NACOSA process had assured that the plurality of HIV and AIDS stakeholders had come on board in 1992 to embark on the design by early 1994 of an ideal national strategy to counter the AIDS epidemic. In Marais' (2000: 13) analysis, the 'ideal' nature of the NAP was the result of the fact that, due to the incipient political transition, consensus was more easily marshalled, debates were polarised into support for the new or support for the old, the influence of organisations and individuals with progressive credentials and histories was strong, and the Plan was drafted more or less in an institutional and fiscal vacuum, unrestrained by the practicalities of governance. 'In this sense', Marais (2000: 13) states, 'it was analogous to the ANC's adoption of the Reconstruction and Development Programme'.

By the time South Africans woke up to the Rainbow Nation on 27 April 1994, the NACOSA National AIDS Plan (NAP) had been drafted and approved by amongst others, policy actors of all the main political parties representing ordinary South Africans. Furthermore, civil society as well as big business had bought into the process, and there were grand hopes that the human rights-centred approach that informed the NAP would bear fruit via swift and effective implementation by a democratic government.

This chapter focuses on the three main phases of AIDS policy making that are discernable during the Mandela administration. During the first phase, from 1994 until early 1996, the Reconstruction and Development Programme (RDP) was held up as the broad public policy blueprint that would improve the country's socio-political equity. The RDP also served as the ideological foundation of other policy measures, including the NAP. However, exactly two years later (in April 1996) the RDP was abandoned and replaced by the fiscally conservative Growth, Employment and Redistribution Programme (GEAR).[1] It was also at that time that the ANC government had to face the reality that – due to an array of implementation difficulties – the NAP had failed to make any significant dent in the country's rapidly expanding AIDS epidemic.

This introduced the second phase of efforts at stemming the advance of the South African AIDS epidemic. Unfortunately the two years immediately following the scrapping of the RDP and the re-evaluation of South Africa's public response to HIV and AIDS were marked by a rapid succession of so-called AIDS scandals and other instances of maladministration: the country lurched from the *Sarafina II* humiliation to the Virodene controversy to the government's wholly bewildering handling of the provision of anti-retroviral drugs to pregnant women.[2] To make

1 Importantly, the ANC government has maintained that it never actually abandoned the RDP and that GEAR was never so much a replacement of the RDP than an additional policy designed to strengthen its developmentalist approach with a focus on economic growth.

2 The transmission of HIV from mother to child (MTCT) is also referred to as the 'vertical' transmission of the virus – from pregnant or birthing mother to child. This occurs

matters worse, the Mandela government then confounded its AIDS critics by unilaterally moving towards making AIDS a notifiable disease – despite the fact that both the original NAP as well as the AIDS elite in South Africa had agreed upon and espoused the opposite policy ideals.

These events worked against a successful third phase of policy making on HIV and AIDS during the Mandela administration, namely, the launch in late 1998 of a renewed cross-sectoral 'Partnership Against AIDS'. Sadly, by that time the epidemic had become endemic to the country, and it had become at least as politicised as it had been under the NP government.

As is outlined in more detail in Part II, the Mandela government's failure to assess, rework and improve the defunct NAP may again point to possible instances of partial acknowledgement. Whilst the contested political environment of the early 1990s could to an extent account for the lack of action on the AIDS-front at the time, the new democratic dispensation's failure to deliver on what it had discussed and planned in so much detail leading up to democratisation, brings the issue into sharp relief. That the NAP overestimated the institutional capacity of the new government goes some way towards explaining their initial lack of response. However, subsequent failures to revise this strategy and to take a renewed proactive response raise suspicions that government's acknowledgement of the AIDS situation was only partial. Whether this was the result of continued institutional incapacity or a matter of political preoccupation will be explored later in this book. The controversies that punctuated the latter part of Mandela's tenure further enforce suspicions of government denial.

The National AIDS Plan of 1994

Idealism versus implementation

As noted in the previous chapter the redefinition of AIDS as a human rights and development issue and its subsequent repositioning on the public agenda led in 1992 to the broadly inclusive 'South Africa united against AIDS' conference. This meeting established NACOSA and was described by AIDS analysts as 'an unusual show of national unity at a time of complex and sensitive political negotiations, well before an election date for a democratically elected government had been decided' (Nattrass 2004: 42). By 1992 the normative AIDS policy environment had shifted away from an exclusive conception of the epidemic as a health policy problem, and now emphasised and embraced the need for a human rights-based approach.

It was this confluence of a changed policy environment, the inclusion of the majority of important AIDS stakeholders and a sense of urgency that led to the

---

at three instances: at the antenatal stage (during pregnancy), during the birth process itself, or post-natally, through the HIV-positive mother's breast milk.

Table 4.1 HIV seroprevalence in South Africa

Year	1990	1991	1992	1993	1994	1995	1996	1997	1998	1999	2000
% of women attending antenatal clinics	0.8	1.4	2.4	4.3	7.6	10.4	14.2	17.0	22.8	22.4	24.5
% of total population	0.1	0.1	0.6	1.1	1.8	2.9	4.5	6.3	8.2	10.1	11.7

Source: Data compiled from Dorrington and Johnson (2002: 34).

drafting of South Africa's first comprehensive public strategy on HIV and AIDS: the National AIDS Plan (NAP) was officially adopted at Cabinet level in October 1994. It was only once political will had come about and was translated into a reconceptualisation of the AIDS policy problem that an appropriate and widely accepted public policy could be drafted. However, in retrospect it is clear that by the end of the Mandela Presidency in June 1999 the NAP policy framework had failed dismally at achieving its goals. The idealism accompanying the ANC's acceptance of the NAP and its human rights approach in April 1994 and the Cabinet's approval of it as the official public policy response to HIV and AIDS in October 1994 was sadly misplaced.

Despite the claim in 1994 that the NAP was an 'ideal' policy that got everything right in terms of inclusiveness, normative underpinnings and human rights-centred policy prescriptions, the empirical data proved otherwise.[3] Table 4.1 above quantifies the unabated growth in AIDS prevalence figures as derived from both antenatal clinic surveys as well as national extrapolations that covered the whole South African population.

The data demonstrates that – in terms of absolute numbers – the NAP was ineffective.[4] It was unable to achieve any AIDS strategy's primary goal: over time to lower HIV prevalence and AIDS-related morbidity and mortality among the population. The HIV prevalence figure among women attending antenatal clinics in 1994 was a disquieting 7.6 per cent, but instead of decreasing or even stabilising as a result of the implementation of the NAP during the Mandela government, this figure more than tripled to 24.5 per cent by the year 2000. Concomitantly, the HIV

3 Reflecting on this idealism, Schneider and Stein (2001: 723) note that '[t]he policy space, defined as "room for manoeuvre and influence" around government appeared wide. The expectation was that enlightened forces in civil society would work together with the new government to steer the rapid implementation of a well-formulated and rights-oriented National AIDS Plan'.

4 Dr Ashraf Grimwood, the one-time chairperson of NACOSA summed this up by saying that 'South Africa's history of addressing AIDS is the most appalling debacle. We have shot our allies, knifed our neighbours, and instead of attacking the enemy, attacked each other' (quoted in Van der Vliet 2004a: 80).

prevalence figure among the population as a whole was 1.8 per cent in 1994, but this figure ballooned by 650 per cent to a national HIV prevalence figure of 11.7 per cent by 2000.

Clearly, something had gone badly wrong. Analysts are in agreement that the contents of the actual NAP strategy could not be faulted. There is wide agreement among policy and AIDS analysts that the NAP had been the result of an ideal policy drafting process. The contents of the actual Plan contained all the elements required by HIV and AIDS and policy stakeholders including the World Health Organisation's (WHO) Global Programme on AIDS (GPA) officials, members of South African civil society, business, political parties, AIDS activists and trade unions.

A more politically correct and seemingly socially appropriate policy could hardly be imagined.[5] The NAP came about during the time of the drafting of the new South Africa's first critical macroeconomic and developmental framework – the RDP. It can be no coincidence that both the RDP and the NAP were accepted by the ANC a few weeks prior to the April 1994 election. Also, the RDP was written in such a manner that it embraced the normative tenets of the NAP, going as far as elevating the NAP as one of its five key elements.[6] Juxtaposing the RDP and the NAP, the numerous congruencies between the two programmes are noteworthy.[7] The ANC's new Health Programme, the RDP as well as the NAP espoused the following values: inclusive, conciliatory, stable and consensual policy making, focusing on bottom-up, populist measures and mechanisms to ensure that the all the appropriate policy stakeholders take ownership of the policies. Marais (1998: 180) referred to the result of these ideals as a nexus of policies that 'established a comfort zone between conflicting forces and interests'.

These so-called 'pro-poor policies' had a strong developmental slant, with goals to embrace social spending for the sake of alleviating the plight of the indigent (Mbali 2003: 313). Initially for example the RDP base document had pledged among other things to:

- Shift the health system from curative services towards primary health care (PHC), with free medical services for children under six years and pregnant

---

5 According to Whiteside and Sunter (2000: 119–20) 'there were major flaws in the NACOSA plan – not in the contents, which are still valid today, but in the lack of attention to process and the failure to acknowledge the realities of the social, political and economic situation in South Africa at the time. In effect, there was no "reality check", a fundamental principle of good planning'.

6 Five Presidential Lead Projects were identified within the RDP and placed under the custodianship of the National Department of Health. The HIV and AIDS and STD Programme was one of these five (Karim 1995: 11). In fact, as the National Department of Health (2000: 6) noted in its Primary Health Care Report in 2000, Mandela referred specifically to HIV and AIDS as one of his key RDP priorities during his inaugural address on 10 May 1994.

7 As Whiteside (1998: 100) said of the NAP, '[t]he overarching national policies, like the RDP, set the framework for national development policies…'.

women at state facilities – by 1998, all South Africans were to receive their basic nutritional intake, thanks to school-feeding and other schemes.
- Create 2.5 million new jobs within ten years.
- Provide electricity to 2.5 million homes by the year 2000, doubling the number of households with such access from the then 36 per cent.
- Provide running water and sewage systems to one million households.
- Provide ten years of free education.
- Extend infrastructure through a public works programme; and
- Restructure state institutions to reflect the racial, class and gender composition of South African society (Marais 1998: 180).

The NAP also reflected the broad policy goals of the RDP by emphasising 'a new division of responsibility for health between the different levels of government' and adopting an intersectoral approach (Price and Van Heerden 1994: 34). The RDP-NAP nexus was so strong that one analyst noted that:

> [t]he rational and logical way properly to manage [AIDS] is to contextualise it within the [RDP] paradigm, and to approach the problem with the principles and concepts embodied in the RDP. The RDP concept itself will in the long run do the most to minimise the impact of the epidemic… (Evian 1995: 3).

The ANC's National Health Plan of May 1994 (ANC 1994: 1) explicitly noted that '[a]ll legislation, organisations and institutions related to health have to be reviewed' with a view to ensuring that the emphasis went beyond the apartheid era's focus on biomedical responses, focusing on health and overall well-being instead. To this end, it was envisaged that a Charter of Patients' Rights would be enacted, placing PHC central to the nation's health. Importantly, Schneider (2001: 3; 2002: 145) refers to the establishment of the AIDS policy process during the early days of the Mandela government as existing in the arena of 'high politics' – on a level where strategies and ideals compete and are established as core values, including national self-preservation, and the long-term objectives of the state. Since AIDS policy making entered this high stakes game at such an early stage, with core statal values underpinning it, it is important to evaluate the changes that appeared later on as macro-policy values and policy agenda items shifted around the year 1996.

Although an in-depth analysis of the contents of actual policies is beyond the ambit of this book, a brief overview of the NAP's key elements is in order (Smart 2002: 190–92).[8] In the first instance, the NAP entailed an integrated response to HIV and AIDS and comprised six elements: education and prevention; counselling; health care; human rights and law reform; welfare, and research. According to Marais (2000: 12–13), key among the principles adopted was that people living

8 For more in-depth discussions of the programmatic contents of the NAP, see Fleming (1994: 9–11), Karim (1995: 11–12), Manning (2001: 42–66) and McKerrow (2002: 177–80).

with HIV and AIDS (PWAs) would be involved in all prevention, intervention and care strategies; that the NAP would be guided by recognition of women's vulnerable position; and that confidentiality would be protected. Importantly, the Plan did not view the epidemic primarily as a medical issue but couched AIDS education, prevention and care in broader, social terms.

As important, the NAP also emphasised the imperative for both prevention and care strategies – in later years, a rather contrived dichotomy between the two aspects would appear in the government's public policy statements (as if HIV and AIDS prevention and care were mutually exclusive). In the NAP, however, all sectors of government were to be enlisted in the fight against AIDS. Thus, the NAP's goal and objects were to:

- Prevent the transmission of HIV.
- Provide care for people infected with and affected by AIDS.
- Alleviate the impact of AIDS on communities.
- Support people not infected by HIV in their efforts to retain that status.
- Provide a forum for all South Africans to become involved in efforts to combat the spread of HIV and AIDS.
- Identify resources that could be deployed in the fight against AIDS; and
- Ensure that communities were fully involved in all stages of the development, planning and implementation of the Plan.

Lastly, implementation would be guided by the pursuit of three, overriding objectives: preventing the spread of HIV; reducing the personal and social impact of HIV and AIDS, and mobilising and unifying national, provincial, international and local resources – again a strong balance between and interlocked system of prevention and care was mooted.

Explaining the failure of the NAP

So what went wrong? Why did this supposedly ideal, near-perfect vision and policy on HIV and AIDS fail to have any impact on the epidemic in South Africa? In Marais' (2000: 6, 8) analysis the policy implementation environment at the time goes some way to explaining this failure:

> [i]n the 1990s South Africa was the only country in the world which had to contend with an exponential rise in HIV prevalence rates in the context of a major political transition. In 1990–94, therefore, what was unavailable was the institutional and political stability – not to mention the political legitimacy of government – necessary to implement a coherent and co-ordinated response…It is widely held that the difficulties encountered [in 1994–99] related to questions of process rather than technical content – hence the emphasis on the contextual problems that hampered implementation.

Remarkably, the reasons offered for the failure of the NAP are almost identical to the explanations pointed to for the *de facto* scrapping of the RDP in April 1996. Taken as a whole, the failure of the NAP can be summed up as suffering from a 'crisis of implementation' – the strategic and operational details of the NAP document simply did not move beyond the problem identification, agenda-setting, policy formulation and policy adoption phases.[9] There were a number of factors that kept the NAP from being effectively operationalised. These factors are important in that they for the most part either were partly the result of the legacy of bad AIDS policy responses during the administration of NP governments, or the specific policy environment introduced issues that would impact negatively on AIDS policy making and implementation in years to come.

The sad irony of the NAP was that what had been projected as one of its most positive features seemed to be the direct antecedent of its downfall (Marais 2000: 15). The purportedly ideal, rather idealistic, programmatic specifications and policy prescriptions of the NAP fell victim to precisely its idealism: the NAP was not realistic in what it wanted to achieve. During the time when the NAP was drafted via the NACOSA process of 1992–94, the ANC had not yet come to power, the white government's power was steadily following the downward spiral of its political authority, and human rights activists in particular could interact with other AIDS policy actors and agents and draw up a strategy in a context wholly divorced from the everyday realities of governance. The NAP came about and was accepted by the ANC caucus in early April 1994 as its main policy strategy to deal with HIV and AIDS before the party was exposed to the harsh realities of government.

The NAP in its original form was thus the expression of a wish-list; the ultimate luxury afforded to policy makers who had been operating outside of the harsh constraints of budget realities and any real consideration for implementation capacity during a time of radical political and institutional transformation. Moreover, there was precious little accountability required of the essentially unelected group who made up NACOSA. The context of 1992–94 meant that the NAP accepted in April 1994 was almost inevitably festooned as a moral script, with serious consideration of whether it was practicable or not left by the wayside. It was the AIDS equivalent of the ANC's Freedom Charter of the 1950s: a document espousing laudable, 'high political' values – the difference being that the NAP gave little thought to the programmatic practicalities that would face its implementers.

Also, one has to bear in mind that the NAP came about during a parallel ideological battle between those in favour of retaining elements of apartheid versus those who wanted to create a wholly transformed society. The progression of the constitutional negotiations being held in Kempton Park at the same time,

9 Friedman (1997: 16) identified implementation as an area of general policy making malaise: '... many of our policy proposals fail to recognise that policy needs to be rooted in the society and ignore the gulf between abstract reasoning and social reality. Only half a policy has been devised if that policy has failed to come to grips with the practicalities and details of implementation'.

and the moral high ground of the constitutional transformationalists (as well as their prowess at the negotiation table) meant that the NAP was couched in a zero-sum moral discourse: one was either for a radically changed approach to combating HIV and AIDS in South Africa, or one remained stuck in the morally discredited AIDS interventions that had been practiced and implemented by the NP government. Given those odds, it is little wonder that the NAP so strongly and unquestioningly embraced the human rights-centred approach and that it had such an idealist slant – without sufficient, realistic thought of counter-ideological arguments, or the constraints of practicalities.

As a result, it can now be said that the new government took on too much.[10] In keeping with the developmental focus of its other flagship macro-policy, the RDP, it became generally understood that the new government would be at the helm of national developmental efforts. It was primarily up to the government to provide to the poor, to change the look and feel of South African society, and to ameliorate societal ills – including HIV and AIDS. In the discursive environment of the RDP and despite lip service to the participation of civil society and the ANC's political alliance partners the government would take on the primary responsibility to improve all South Africans' quality of life. The ideological idealism of this position is less important than the immense pressure on and role that it presupposed for the South African state.

It might be that the ANC's most central mistake in the first few years of its coming to power was its overpowering urge to improve all of South Africa; to be everything for everyone. Instead of focusing on a handful of governance or policy issues in which it could make a realistic, considered difference, the new government aimed to do justice to the spirit underlying the Mandela era: to provide 'a better life for all'. One of the members of NACOSA, Helen Schneider (quoted in Marais 2000: 32), echoes this sentiment, stating that:

> [i]n retrospect, one of the problems with the NACOSA process was that it loaded too much on government's shoulders – there was a belief that things would just happen much more effectively than they did. In a way we couldn't have done better at the time, but there should have been a rapid process of reviewing, a constant process of assessing and asking questions. That didn't really happen, not even within government.

The implications of such a government-centred mindset are twofold. On the one hand, the world of AIDS activism would welcome such an approach, since it presupposes the critically important strong political ownership of the AIDS problem (which purportedly had worked particularly well in Uganda under President Museveni) (AIDS Analysis Africa 1995: 1). On the other hand, however, some analysts point out that this places too much of a burden and responsibility on the government.

---

10 According to Schrire (2001: 22) '[s]ome of this was probably inevitable. People expected far more from Mbeki than any government could have delivered'.

The primarily sexual nature of HIV transmission means that any grand societal behaviour modification needs to happen at the individual, coital level – and no government can realistically or successfully take overall responsibility for individuals' sexual behaviour (Ainsworth 1999: 107) – in fact, such a political proclivity would come dangerously close to trying to govern the grey area between what is 'public' and what is 'private'. As noted in the discussion on the apartheid years, under the NP government there had been broad policies aimed at policing sexual mixing, much to the antipathy of human rights and anti-apartheid activists all over the world. The new government was adamant that it would not repeat those mistakes, yet its adoption of the NAP and the statements surrounding what government hoped it would achieve meant that the state was setting itself up for failure – and attack.[11]

There were four key sets of resources that the new government could employ in combating AIDS. These included: government officials, existing public structures and institutions aimed specifically at reducing the spread and impact of AIDS, fiscal resources (public money), as well as the newly established context of co-operation between government and civil society.

In the first place, the new government was the result of and institutionally supported by a so-called 'sunset clause' negotiated during the Kempton Park process. Marais (1998: 87) notes that the clause:

> provid[ed] for a period of compulsory power-sharing in the form of the GNU, an offer not to purge the security forces and civil service of 'counter-revolutionary' elements, and the willingness to establish (during negotiations) a set of Constitutional Principles that could not be violated by the final Constitution.

This meant that civil servants who had served under the NP government would not lose their jobs for five years. In other words, the new government was in the fortunate position that – although the ANC had no experience of governing South Africa – it had a cohort of experienced policy implementers at its disposal. In theory, this opened up an opportunity for the new government to make use of existing expertise (also on HIV and AIDS) residing in its public sector and to use this resource in order to drive the implementation of the NAP. However, this supposed resource proved to be a double-edged sword: many of the public sector workers who had served under the NP were now either paralyzingly unsure of their own positions, leading to low overall morale and productivity, or plainly unwilling to assist their new colleagues and new political masters in effectively implementing the NAP.

One explanation for this could be the reported bitterness amongst some existing civil servants about having to hierarchically vacate comfortable positions and train their former 'enemies' in the liberation movements in the skills of governance

---

11 According to Schneider and Stein (2001: 727) the call 'for more involvement by politicians can…be a double-edged sword and can be interpreted as the need to "take control"'. 'Politicians have their own imperatives and objectives, and could be caricatured as not seeing beyond the next election' (Schneider 1998: 8).

(Marais 2000: 16). Unfortunately, there was also an explanation focusing on racism: that the white 'old guard', due to their own racism, were tacitly refusing to co-operate fully with the black 'new guard', in the process making the state impotent in its efforts to implement the NAP as well as other public initiatives.

The idealism of the NAP process thus did not find sufficient application in the actual implementation capacity expected of the new government – this capacity had been taken for granted, but now failed to pay off.[12] It became clear that the GNU would have to learn to muddle through with AIDS only one amongst an array of pressing issues on the public agenda (Dorrington and Johnson 2002: 22). These difficulties at the personal level of public sector work compounded the possibility of the new government making effective use of the existing public institutions that had been established to combat the AIDS epidemic.

Chief amongst these bodies were the ATICS – ready-made AIDS centres in urban (mostly white) areas with solid experience and resources to provide some level of both preventative as well as treatment input to ordinary South Africans. The ATICS were all but abandoned by the GNU – they were viewed as belonging to the apartheid era, and reflecting the values of that time (Van der Vliet 2004b: 49; Joseph 2002: 30–31). Also, 'the popular perception of the ATICS, shared by many in the ANC, was that they were staffed mainly by gay and white liberals' (*Washington Post*, 14 July 2000). Unfortunately the demise of the ATICS meant that the government, in addition to losing these institutional structures, also lost the human capital that the ATICS had enabled: the corporate memory, skills and the people employed there (Manning 2001: 62).

These individual and institutional level constraints were exacerbated by the transformation process underway inside the state: South Africa prior to 1994 had one central government and four provincial administrations, but in the democratic dispensation after 1994 the state had to adapt to a new unitary government (incorporating the former apartheid 'homelands'), as well as nine provinces.[13] In addition to the institutional and procedural headaches that this implied, it soon

12 Some analysts point to the WHO's participation in the NACOSA process as one of the factors hindering later implementation of the NAP. The WHO's Global Programme on AIDS (GPA) sent technical advisers to help develop an implementation strategy, but these advisers had little or no experience in South Africa (Winsbury 1994: 3; AIDS Analysis Africa 1994: 2). The GPA's input has been criticised for (1) treating all of Africa as homogeneous in terms of policy needs, (2) their NAP implementation strategy would be too expensive, (3) it presupposed too vast a role for the newly established provincial governments, and assumed a level of capacity at the local government level that was not based on reality, and (4) lastly, South Africans taking part in the NACOSA process lacked the confidence to counter the input of these 'experts' (Crewe 1999: 30).

13 As Crewe (2000: 29) points out, '[t]he failure to implement the Plan stems in part from the political settlement in 1994, which allowed for a national government and nine provincial governments, making it possible to have 10 different policies in key areas. There are in effect 10 different AIDS plans, as each province vies for autonomy and control. What this has meant is that much energy has been spent in feuding and in arguments over

became apparent that the 'GNU' was an institutional misnomer: there was very little effective communication between the central government and the various provincial governments, but in addition the new mechanisms for the devolution of powers and responsibilities were untested and – in the first few years of the existence of the new government – this implied little effective central-provincial co-ordination (Badcock-Walters 2002: 108).

The effect of this on the public battle against HIV and AIDS was that there was an overall impotence in the public sector, with the provincial governments left twisting in a policy vacuum: not only did they rarely receive enough money in their individual health budgets (Schneider and McIntyre 1994: 14; Strachan 1995: 2; Strachan 1996: 322); they increasingly appeared to lack the capacity to spend the AIDS funds that they had. Despite the fact that the NAP received relatively limited funding – certainly below what was required to implement the Plan effectively – Schneider (1998: 5) noted that '[f]rom 1994 to 1997 the AIDS programme consistently underspent on its allocated budget'. Whiteside and Sunter (2000: 120) echo this sentiment, noting that 'the NACOSA budget was R257 million, more than ten times the 1994 national AIDS budget. Even if the funds had been available, the human resources were not and it would never have been possible to meet the targets in the Plan'.

Little co-ordination of human capital at different levels of government meant that the state's capacity to implement an effective AIDS policy became even more of a fiction. Increasingly, the GNU was centralising the governance of health and other public sectors. The first sign of this was the fact that the ANC government, instead of situating the NAP in the office of the Head of State for the sake of urgent implementation and overall checks and balances (as had been agreed upon in the NAP), established an HIV and AIDS and STD Directorate inside the National Department of Health.[14] According to Marais (2000: 10, 11), the original NAP had envisaged that:

> AIDS was to be transported beyond the realm of medicine and converted into a social and political issue. Simultaneously, in terms of treatment, services and an ultimate cure, it was still lodged in the medical field. The one area of action was the expanse of broader society; the other was a district of specialised expertise. Straddling these two realms was the belief that rational behaviour would halt the epidemic's spread…What still eludes us is how to merge the paradigms of the

---

ownership, policy and programmes, rather than in looking for a shared vision and policy and programme developments'.

14 The staff structure of the directorate was only finalised in the 1996/97 financial year (Strode and Smart 1996: 10–11). By 1998 it could draw on only 18 staff members and seven short-term consultants. In addition, the combined provincial/district staffing for AIDS varied 'from 6 to 24 professionals, many of whom ha[d] tasks other than AIDS or STDs' (Schneider 1998: 3). (For a discussion of the difficulties experienced at the region/district level in particular, see Galloway (1996: 7–9)).

> medical and the political, the scientific and the social. There have been attempts to do so, but flawed ones...[T]he Plan was prevented from attaining its goals by incomplete understandings of the social, cultural and ideological terrains on which it had to work.

Situating the governance of AIDS in the National Department of Health thus undermined a critical goal of the NAP: to change the conception of the AIDS problem away from being a public health issue and establishing it as a developmental and human rights issue.[15] In effect, this let the office of the Presidency off the hook: although Mandela had paid lip service to making HIV and AIDS a central part of his Presidential lead projects, the Minister of Health would (once again) become the main institutional custodian of the state's battle against AIDS.[16]

> [T]he location of the Plan in the Department of Health highlighted the tension between the medical and social understandings of HIV and AIDS. The emphasis would be on the biomedical, behaviourist model of health intervention. This model hinges on aiding and persuading individuals to make certain behavioural choices *despite* the constraints created by social status. It is an approach that avoids looking at the complex social transactions people perform in order to position themselves as advantageously as possible in society. Essentially, it is a rationalist approach that sees behaviour as the outcome of transparent predictable and consistent decisions that can be altered by new, equally rational, inputs. Applied to HIV and AIDS it runs into two problems: HIV and AIDS are a disease that seems to defy rationality, and the approach shows a profound lack of knowledge and understanding of stressed social behaviour (Marais 2000: 15).

Significantly, this undermined the relationship between South Africa's HIV and AIDS civil society and the government, and counteracted the spirit underpinning the NAP's mission to facilitate inter- and cross-sectoral co-operation. Instead of taking on the AIDS issue at a macro yet powerful Presidential level, it was left up to the health and other individual government departments to co-ordinate

---

15 Nattrass (2004: 43) points out that this repositioning was accompanied by the allocation of fairly junior civil servants: 'provincial-level AIDS managers were drawn at fairly low levels of seniority from the ranks of the old civil service and were given the task of implementing a programme through weak district structures over which they had no direct line of authority'. Also, see Lush and Makoala (1999: 21).

16 Jeter (2000: 5) notes that '[e]ven the revered Mandela made no public mention of AIDS until he delivered a speech in late 1997 to the World Health Organization, and that was in Switzerland. His first public remarks on the subject in South Africa were not spoken until 1998, more than three years into his Presidency'. In later years, Mandela cited his handling of HIV and AIDS during his Presidency as a major failure of his administration (*The Star*, 4 March 2003).

activities.[17] The distance that had grown between the government and civil society on this issue was later played out in the discursive environment and AIDS actors' willingness and ability to redefine the AIDS policy problem – as discussed below, the schism between civil society and the state presaged a battle between the government's increasingly obdurate position on the importance of prevention versus civil society's insistence on access to treatment for people who were already living with the virus.

The Health Department under the new Minister of Health, Dr Nkosazana Zuma (ex-wife of current South African President Jacob Zuma), and the government as a whole did not respond well to criticism of this and other stances. An increasingly intransigent Health Minister either insisted on loyalty to the transformation process in South Africa – deeming any questioning of or negative comment on her department's actions on HIV and AIDS as either party-politically disloyal, or racist (particularly in the case of media criticism).[18] Such obduracy foreshadowed the further deterioration of the relationship between the HIV and AIDS civil society and the Health Minister and government, in effect re-politicising and re-racialising AIDS. A siege mentality had developed within the government, and it soon became a permanent feature of the gamut of the AIDS policy pathology. As Nattrass (2004: 44) points out:

> [i]nstead of acting quickly and efficiently to solve the implementation problems, South Africa's political leadership initially engaged in disastrous high profile 'quick fix' solutions. When these failed, and as HIV prevalence increased, the government went on the defensive by questioning the cost-effectiveness and affordability of AIDS interventions requiring the use of antiretrovirals.

Summarising the contextual issues that worked against the effective implementation of the NAP, Schneider (1998: 7–8) notes the following as key issues:

- The delayed development of programme infrastructure at both national and provincial level post-1994.
- The lack of experience of new cadres in policy implementation through a large bureaucracy (as opposed to project implementation through NGOs) combined with a culture of non-delivery inherited from the old structures.

---

17 Deputy President Mbeki did, however, on 8 October 1997 announce in Parliament that the Cabinet had approved the establishment of an Inter-Departmental Committee on AIDS (IDC), which he would chair (Hatane 1999: 12).

18 An incident illustrating this mindset took place a few years into the Mandela administration, when Health Minister Zuma – frustrated by the Director of the Medical Control Council's (MCC) refusal to approve the ARV drug Virodene – rounded on him: 'You're ANC. Why won't you back me on this?' (quoted in Van der Vliet 2004b: 56). Van der Vliet (2004b: 57) continues to say that '[g]iven that the media, the opposition parties and the leadership of many in AIDS organizations were white, it was perhaps inevitable that [Minister Zuma] translated criticism against herself into a counter-charge of racism – a charge which in turn drew anger and derision from blacks in the field'.

- The inability of a state undergoing restructuring at every level to prioritise AIDS in the face of multiple other, more visible priorities.
- Failure to capitalise on infrastructure developed prior to 1994.
- Implementation too narrowly focused on health sector rather than cross-sectorally as recommended by the Plan.
- Weakening of NGOs by the loss of leadership to government/state structures.
- Difficulties in defining and co-ordinating roles and responsibilities between different levels of an evolving federal system; and
- Conflict between stakeholders around unilateral policy development by senior government officials, and the lack of consultation with, and representation from, the broader AIDS community.[19]

In addition, the NAP itself had the following weaknesses: it was a detailed blueprint for implementation developed prior to a massive change in the political and overall policy environment. With the exception of one provincial AIDS co-ordinator, the core members of the task teams who drafted the Plan did not lead its implementation post-1994. Seven of the nine provincial co-ordinators were not involved in the process at all. Institutional or policy making memory became lost, as was ownership of the Plan. Furthermore, it focused on the technical content of policy, but did not pay sufficient attention to processes of policy implementation, in particular how various actors could come together to support implementation. Also, it relied too much on government rather than on mobilising the multiplicity of actors outside of government – as Schneider (2002: 163) notes:

> calls for political leadership not only place an inappropriate emphasis on the agency of national political leaders, but also project them as always willing and able to take the best possible courses of action to address the problems of HIV.

These challenges to implementing the NAP go a long way to contextualising South Africa's inaction in the period directly following democratisation in 1994. This overview also sketches a context that is essential to arguments around the government's partial acknowledgement of the epidemic that are expounded later in this discussion. Implementation of the NAP was clearly fraught with difficulties. But whilst the failure of this idealistic strategy was tragic, its shortcomings pointed the way for a dramatic restructuring of South Africa's AIDS policy. It is government's subsequent failure to consider the valuable lessons that were contained in the NAP's foundering that bolsters our argument for possible official denial during this period.

---

19 'Reflective of the style of governance in the National Department of Health, the then Minister of Health commented that "AIDS does not consult, it infects people"'(Schneider 2002: 147).

A comedy of errors

Despite the quantifiable failure of the NAP it was not abandoned or even amended. Instead there was a national review of South Africa's response to the AIDS epidemic that was published in mid-1997. The review was entitled *Review the Past, Plan the Future, Work Together* and contained very few surprises relating to government's broad AIDS policy prescriptions. The review findings highlighted the need for:

- Political leadership and public commitment.
- Meaningful involvement of people living with HIV and AIDS in policy formulation.
- Responses to be interdepartmental and intersectoral.
- Widespread capacity building.
- Close co-operation with the TB Programme; and
- An urgent address of human rights abuses and the reduction of stigmatisation (Whiteside and Sunter 2000: 122; Ngwena and Pelser 2001: 4).

In short, the review contained nothing really new and very few additions that would point to any shift regarding HIV and AIDS. It merely reiterated the spirit and the letter of the original NAP of 1994. Due to the stated 'ideal' nature of the original NAP, this is hardly surprising – why would any government tinker with the contents of a programme that enjoyed the buy-in of all the main AIDS policy stakeholders? The most glaring error of the 1997 review was the fact that it repeated the key mistake of the NAP: to ignore the actual AIDS policy environment. Instead of a short-term revision of the NAP or any profound evaluation of its implementation difficulties the National Department of Health started to do exactly the opposite: they shifted in emphasis from implementation to devising guidelines, with the stated goal to develop capacity and improve co-ordination (Marais 2000: 22).

By that stage however the broader policy environment itself had shifted: in April 1996 the government announced that the RDP office would be closed. Despite the government's reassurances that the developmental focus of its main policy documents would not be abandoned, the ANC in power opted instead to maintain more of a distance from the programmatic practicalities required of its pro-poor policy history. In the place of the RDP, the GEAR strategy was to be the new macroeconomic keystone of the government. This programme, announced in June 1996 after remarkably little co-ordination amongst the broader corporatist policy environment as well as little consultation with the ANC's main political alliance partners, would lead to an exponential rise in the power of the Ministry of Finance in determining spending priorities in the affairs of state, as well as determining actual policy priorities. This has important implications: the pro-poor values and developmental policy slant of the RDP would make way for a much more financially conservative, 'Washington consensus'-based model.

The ANC in government thus moved from a pro-poor policy making stance to a pro-growth macroeconomic policy stance – with the latter couched in the discursive environment of employment creation and low budget deficits. The low social spending implied by such a macroeconomic policy shift had maybe the greatest impact on the critically important health sector. Instead of prioritising spending on social and health services, the government's policy discourse now changed to one of combating dissaving (as spending on social services would be viewed) and emphasising fiscal discipline rather than tolerance for budget deficits. This move foreshadowed a significant institutional shift – in terms of HIV and AIDS policy making and spending priorities, it lead to the tacit re-definition (yet again) of the AIDS policy problem, which would become much clearer a few years later: the monetarisation of AIDS.

The first phase of public policy making on HIV and AIDS under the Mandela government effectively came to an end in the course of 1996. Indicators of the shift to a second phase of AIDS public policy making include: the demonstrable failure to effectively implement the NAP of 1994; the move from the RDP (abandoned in April 1996) to GEAR (announced in June 1996), and the emergence of an AIDS policy environment defined by public scandal.

Not counting the failure on the part of the government to implement the NAP, there were four so-called AIDS policy scandals or polemics in the years between 1994 and 1999. These include *Sarafina II* in 1996; Virodene in 1997; the AZT decision of 1998, and the gradual move on the part of the government away from an entrenchment of the human rights-centred HIV confidentiality principle, to making AIDS notifiable. An a number of occasions official's actions and reactions during these 'scandals' resound with forms of official denial that are contained in Cohen's typology. This is explored more closely below.

Sarafina II

The first scandal to hit the AIDS policy environment of the new government was the so-called *Sarafina II* debacle. In the 1970s and 1980s the South African playwright Mbongeni Ngema came to prominence with his anti-apartheid stage productions. Amongst these was a play (and later a musical filmed and starring the Oscar-winning American actress Whoopi Goldberg) called *Sarafina*, which told the story of a young girl from Soweto and her and her peers' struggle for political freedom. The play and the movie were very popular internationally, emblemising apartheid's dying days.

In 1995 the National Department of Health put out a tender for the production of a stage play with the aim of informing young people across South Africa about the dangers of HIV and AIDS. After meeting with Ngema, senior health officials awarded a R14.27 million tender to the playwright to produce such a stage production. Despite the fact that this amount of money constituted a significant portion of the national AIDS budget, the Minister of Health fast-tracked Ngema's appointment and this led to criticism from the official opposition in Parliament as well as from the white-owned media that the correct tendering procedures had not been followed.[20] In addition, AIDS activists questioned the wisdom of the play's (now entitled *Sarafina II*) central messages, deeming it inappropriate and ineffectual (Parker 1996: 15). One of the main objections that the South African AIDS civil society had was that they were not consulted as to the contents of the play (Zuma 1996: 2).

There were thus two sets of criticism against *Sarafina II*: the contents of the play and its key messages were attacked for falling short of reaching the stated target market (undercutting its value) and the political opposition and the media pointed out that regular tendering processes had not been followed and questioned the amount of money awarded to Ngema. As Kitching (1996: 40) noted:

> [t]he Minister of Health ...cannot justify spending R14.2 million – one fifth of the already limited national Budget and more than the total provincial budgets – on fighting AIDS. Further efforts by the Minister and her Director-General, Dr Olive Shisana, to justify this has also led to a political crisis of morality [translated from Afrikaans].

Other critics were even less kind, with Eichbaum (1996: 3) noting that:

> when the Department of Health embarks upon a R14.27 million exercise to fund a single stage production mounted by a person with an established track record of overspending on mediocrity and, in the process, sidestepping every known convention and procedure for the awarding of such a contract, one's hackles must inevitably rise.

In the months following the mention of these concerns, government's relationship with civil society as well as the opposition and the media rapidly deteriorated. The sad irony was that the AIDS civil society in South Africa was for the most part comprised of former ANC and other anti-apartheid activists. The breakdown of relations between the government and civil society thus came down to a clash within the former broad South African liberation alliance. As the government's opposition to the questioning of the wisdom of *Sarafina II* increased, so did AIDS service organisations become increasingly involved in the politicisation of the issue.

In the process, Crewe (2000: 30) noticed the entrenchment of a politically dangerous stance: the creation of an 'AIDS orthodoxy' inside government (in the National Department of Health in particular) with anything falling outside of that 'orthodoxy' deemed as counter-transformationalist, disloyal or even racist. These

20 Phila (1996: 1–4) noted that '[t]he Public Protector's report spells out clearly that Sarafina II was the idea of Minister Zuma...The Tender Committee objected to some of the line items in the [proposed] budget and did not make a decision. Without the approval of the State Tender Board, the contract...was signed on 10 August 1995...'. The tendering procedures used were not those sanctioned by the Tender Committee, but their forms were used.

accusations relate strongly to what Cohen (2001: 112) terms counter-offensive denial – where officials create leverage in a challenging situation by constructing critics as enemies. This is explored in further detail in Chapter 8. The danger of such a stance is that the AIDS policy environment became a new terrain of high political struggle, with various policy actors and agents within that environment vying for the 'right' to make statements regarding the epidemic – going as far as fighting each other for the right to define the very policy problem itself (Walker, Reid and Cornell 2004: 107).

Health Minister Zuma assumed a particularly combative position, citing racism on the part of the media and opposition parties when they deigned to question or criticise the Department of Health's actions. In particular, Zuma accused her detractors that they were abusing the technical details of a tendering process, pointing to that issue mainly due to the fact that the tender had gone to a black person (Marais 2000: 36). A year later, President Mandela referred to the *Sarafina II* affair as one of the main failings of his Presidency (Nattrass 2004: 45). In the end, the play was never produced, and government wrote off its expenses as to its production years later – under the Mbeki Presidency. Importantly, though, *Sarafina II* embodied a divorce between government and AIDS civil society from which South Africa is yet to recover. As Phila (1996: 4) notes:

> [The *Sarafina II* storm] has left much political and economic damage in its wake for the department [of health] and the young democracy. The credibility of Minister Zuma and senior Department officials has been severely damaged…The policy work of the department was put on hold as this controversy unfolded… Further, the reluctance of some members of the health portfolio committee and Parliament to ask difficult questions of the Ministry of Health during its investigations raises serious questions about the role of Parliament in ensuring transparency and accountability within government.

The combative posturing of both the National Department of Health as well as civil society meant that the shared vision of the NACOSA process two years earlier had all but died. *Sarafina II* introduced and solidified a defensiveness in the government, henceforth rendering AIDS policy making reactive rather than visionary or pro-active. Importantly, analysts would refer to this saga as the birth of 'anti-intellectual' AIDS governance in South Africa – this approach ran counter to the 'pro-knowledge stance' of extra-governmental AIDS activism in South Africa (Schneider 2002: 158) and would become a feature of the public management of the epidemic until the end of the first Mbeki administration in September 2008.

Virodene

The next polemic to make headlines was the government's championing in 1997 of the purported anti-AIDS drug Virodene. The latter was developed by scientists attached to the University of Pretoria, and was touted as a home-grown 'miracle cure' for AIDS. However, despite the fact that the drug had not passed the Medical Control Council's (MCC) clinical trials (Galloway 1999: 21) the Minister of Health facilitated a meeting between the scientists and Cabinet, with the government giving the Virodene scientists a standing ovation at the end of their presentation. Then Deputy President Mbeki himself got involved in the saga by publicly pushing for the MCC's fast-tracking of the drug's approval.[21]

Given the political sensitivities following on from the recent history of *Sarafina II*, the reaction of opposition parties and the South African media was predictable: great opposition to the government's blatant interference in an epistemic community (biomedical science) where they did not belong. To make matters worse the media claimed that the ANC had a financial stake in Virodene's development – emphasising vested party-political interests. The MCC deemed the drug as not sufficiently tested in clinical trials and declared it unfit for human consumption. The MCC was able to demonstrate that Virodene was in fact a derivative of an industrial solvent, dimenthylfomamide (DMF). This 'independent' medical control body was then lambasted by the Minister of Health and eventually (in 1998) disbanded and reconstituted by the National Health Department. The Minister of Health's reaction seemed to suggest that it was in fact that MCC that was hampering government response to the epidemic, and not key officials who were pushing for an industrial solvent to be approved as an AIDS treatment. When the rhetoric that emerged during the Virodene saga is cast against Cohen's typology, it could be considered a form of interpretive official denial.

The Virodene saga is significant in that it opened up the government to a new line of criticism regarding its handling of HIV and AIDS as a public policy issue, namely that the government was interfering in science and not focusing on what they were supposed to be doing: governing the country and implementing policies. Critics pointed out that the National Department of Health rode roughshod over established scientific principles such as peer review and other procedural guidelines, pushing for the drug to be given to humans despite the fact that its clinical trials had not gone beyond the superficial first phase level. Criticism from the opposition Democratic Party (DP) and the South African media of the reported financial stake that the governing party had in the development of Virodene was countered by allegations of racism. The Minister of Health went as far as to intimate that the opposition wanted black people to die and hence was opposed to any possible solution to the AIDS epidemic.[22] Again, this reaction exhibited elements of counter-offensive official denial (see Chapter 8).

---

21 In Jeter's (2000: 6) analysis, '[t]he Cabinet…believed the discovery would validate South Africa's black majority in much the same way that Christiaan Barnard's first successful heart transplant in 1968 affirmed apartheid South Africa to the world'.

22 Jeter (2000: 6) reports that, '[w]hen the opposition Democratic Party criticized the ANC's endorsement of Virodene, Zuma responded "The DP hates ANC supporters. If they had their way we would all die of AIDS"'.

Instead of focusing on the clinical properties of Virodene and rather than respecting scientific due process the AIDS policy environment was racialised and politicised once again.

The irony of the history of Virodene was that the same government and the same prominent Deputy President who was pushing for its registration as an AIDS drug were discounting scientists' and other critics' position that the drug was toxic. Mbeki would in the next year as well as in later years use the very same argument against the wholesale provision of AIDS drugs such as AZT and Nevirapene (even though these drugs had been clinically proven to be effective) (AIDS Analysis Africa 1995b: 8). Again, this underscores the deepening willingness on the part of very senior government officials to insist on monopolising the right to define the AIDS policy problem itself, discounting any position that countered their AIDS orthodoxy. As a result the combative stances of the government and the broader 'AIDS world' in South Africa were further entrenched.

Within the context of *Sarafina II*, this meant that any constructive engagement amongst the actors that constituted the broader AIDS policy community became increasingly impossible. The government blamed all outside of the state that their arguments were based on short-sighted racism, whilst the AIDS civil society found an easy policy scapegoat in the hardening governmental position – the spirit of NACOSA was now truly dead and buried, with no one taking responsibility for combating HIV. Instead of opposing a virus the AIDS community in South Africa was in effect at war with itself. The site of the struggle for a new South Africa had moved from apartheid to AIDS, but the same activists who had fought with the incumbent government against apartheid were now antagonistic to their former comrades.

The National Department of Health and the Office of the Deputy President had touted Virodene as a possible African solution to an African problem, but they ended up with proverbial egg on their faces. Instead of owning up to the fact that it was not in their expertise or interest to 'play science' the government's anti-intellectual stance deepened and soon the media, opposition parties and AIDS activists pointed to the government's mismanagement of the AIDS epidemic as being symptomatic of a general failure on the part of the ANC to govern effectively (*Finansies en Tegniek* 13 September 1996).[23] Of course, the greatest disservice of all of this was done to the fight against AIDS itself – not to mention PWAs (Busse 1995: 22). The government increasingly demonstrated a willingness to want to define the AIDS problem without consulting any other stakeholders and in the

23 Malan (1999: 30–31) notes that AIDS had become symbolic of South African society's need to hold the public sector and senior government officials accountable: 'It made us a society that gave the responsibility for AIDS to politicians, rather than to our nation as a whole…In a way AIDS had become a metaphor for everything that is wrong…' [translated from Afrikaans]. For fascinating discussions of the social construction of HIV and AIDS as a metaphor for broader societal ills, see Sontag (2002: 89–180) and Treichler (1999: 315–29).

search for a quick fix solution to the epidemic arrogant mistakes were made.[24] Unfortunately Mbeki's own enthusiasm to question the science of AIDS did not stop there; the government had not taken the lessons of Virodene to heart.

Not that the government got everything wrong. Although it criticised the state's handling of AIDS policy implementation, the National Health Review of mid-1997 noted great successes in the public sector's management of sexually transmitted infections (STIs) in general. In addition to the factors noted above, the review was however explicit in censuring the government for their centralised manner of decision making. It was clear though that the National Department of Health did not see itself as an equal partner with other actors in the AIDS field (as had been foreseen in the NAP of 1994) and the state as a result remained for the most part closed to criticism. This led Crewe (2000: 31) to observe that, although the Review was critical of the government's AIDS management and policy implementation, the NAP remained in place, it was not amended and the recommendations of the review were never implemented. It is no surprise therefore that the AIDS policy environment at the time was defined by an escalation of distrust and general belligerence amongst policy actors.

The AZT decision

The third main area of AIDS policy contention during the Mandela administration appeared on the public agenda in late 1998, when the government through the National Department of Health announced that it would not provide AZT to HIV-positive pregnant women. AZT had recently, in clinical trials held in Thailand and elsewhere, been proven to be effective in limiting the vertical mother-to-child transmission (MTCT) of HIV (Van der Linde 1999: 16). The government's decision was therefore directly counter to the information provided by science, the spirit of the NACOSA process, as well as the letter of the NAP of 1994. At first the government provided monetary justifications as their main reason for ceasing the provision of AZT to combat MTCT – it was, they stated, simply not cost-effective to purchase high-cost drugs in order to apply them with limited efficacy. The Ministry of Finance supposedly did cost-benefit analyses and came to the conclusion that it would be unaffordable to provide AZT on a large scale. This reasoning was immediately questioned by economists with expertise in such costings (Cowlin 1999: 17), who provided solid evidence to the contrary, namely that it would in fact be more expensive in the longer run not to implement MTCT programmes by providing AZT to pregnant women (Marais 2000: 39).

For instance, in 1998 the MRC published a report stating that:

24 Grundlingh (1999: 60) sums up the dynamics of these 'blame politics' by asking the following rhetorical questions: 'Should the victim, who became infected because of behaviour, be blamed – thus absolving the state of social institutions from responsibility for creation social conditions in which AIDS flourished? Or should the "system" be blamed – thereby exculpating the individual?'.

- An estimated 64,398 paediatric HIV infections occurred from MTCT in South Africa in 1997.
- This represents 11 per cent of the estimated global total.
- Approximately 37 per cent of these might be prevented through a national programme which includes short-course AZT.
- The estimated total cost of the national programme is around R164 million.
- This is equivalent to less than one per cent of the national health budget; and
- Therefore a national programme to reduce MTCT of HIV infection in South Africa would be an affordable, cost-effective and potentially cost-saving public health intervention (Wilkinson and Gilks 1999: 15).

According to Nattrass (2004: 47–8):

> [t]he health ministry persisted with this discourse of unaffordability despite medical and economic research showing that the costs of MTCTP were more than offset by the cost-savings associated with reduced numbers of HIV-related paediatric cases. Nono Simelela, Chief Director (HIV and AIDS and STDs) in the Department of Health, argued…that those advocating MTCTP programmes were 'cherry-picking' and that this was a 'luxury' that the health ministry could not afford as it had to respond to the health needs of all South Africans. In other words, the concern was that money spent on MTCTP was money lost to other parts of the health sector.

In addition it became known that the government and the Department of Health in particular were not actually able to spend their existing health budget (including the MTCT component).[25] The state's argument that it could not afford the implementation of its MTCT programme did not, therefore, hold water – and this fallacy was quantifiable. Detractors of the government's position were doubly justified in their position: in the first instance, economists could prove that the affordability excuse was spurious and in the second place they also exposed the government's inability to spend its existing health budgets. As there is quantifiable evidence to disprove government's monetary argument, this position can quite confidently be classified as a form of official denial. More specifically, this appears to be an example of implicatory official denial by appeals to necessity (see Chapter 7). When it appeared that the government could not prove their case based on the monetarisation of priorities their justification for their decision on AZT changed

25 The *Financial Mail* (14 June 1996: 44–5) reported that '[t]he ANC-dominated [Parliamentary health] committee has broken ranks with the organisation's leadership by responding tersely to the *Sarafina II* debacle and criticising the department's failure to implement that national HIV and AIDS prevention programme. Only R2m out of the R13m budget has been spent'.

yet again: the affordability argument was replaced by the National Department of Health questioning the efficacy and the safety of the drug itself.

In fact, the Health Department started to attack the merits of the drug on grounds of toxicity, stating that it would be irresponsible for them to provide AZT to HIV-positive women. Significantly, this was the same government that less that a year before had discounted scientific proof of the toxicity of Virodene in an effort to bypass peer review and other biomedical processes to register a home-grown quick fix to the South African AIDS epidemic. The difference with AZT however was the fact that it had been proven effective by completed international peer reviewed clinical trials. Again the government questioned the science of AIDS despite evidence to the contrary. And again, this is very likely to have been another case of interpretive official denial. We explore this in more detail in Chapter 7.

The monetary arguments used by the government as a whole and the Finance as well as the Health Departments in particular to justify their decision on the non-provision of AZT are significant. Marxists would point to the nexus of exploitation between those elements who own the means to produce a good that is to be used by society as a whole and governments' co-option by these capitalist forces. In the case of the Mandela government's early management of MTCT technologies (the drugs), however, the government itself used Marxian rationalisation for their policy decision. For instance, when it became clear that government was unable to effectively implement public policy on MTCT, the politics of blame resurfaced.

The manner in which it resurfaced was played out as follows: in the first place, government cited the unaffordability of seminal AIDS drugs as a reason not to provide AZT. Instead of owning up to the figures demonstrating the state's actual underspending of its AIDS budget, the government attempted to quantify the (in)affordability of AZT and then disingenuously used Marxian arguments by blaming large pharmaceutical companies and their ownership of the intellectual property rights (IPRs) of ARVs in an effort to apportion ultimate responsibility to these nefarious outside (capitalist) forces. This is an important point, since it would become a major feature of the Mbeki government's handling of the AIDS epidemic in years to come. As this argument became more elaborate during Mbeki's tenure, it began to fit ever more snugly with Cohen's conception of counter-offensive denial (see Chapter 8).

As a consequence, the South African government – as did the NP government before them – turned to AIDS governance via legislation in order to operationalise policy documents. The National Department of Health in 1997 passed the *Medicines and Related Substances Control Amendment Act* (the 'Medicines Act') enabling them to parallel import ARVs from third countries instead of paying what the government called 'exorbitant' fees to large pharmaceutical firms in exchange for drugs. In addition to parallel imports the legislation enabled the government to activate compulsory licensing, which would transfer pharmaceutical technologies to local manufacturers, making it cheaper to produce ARVs locally (Bond 2001: 156).

These measures were entirely legal in terms of International Law and in accordance with World Trade Organisation (WTO) specifications, but were challenged by the large pharmaceutical companies, who decided to take the government to court. The matter became a political hot potato for US Vice-President Al Gore, who around that time was running for office. In the end the pharmaceutical companies withdrew their case against the South African government and unilaterally offered to lower prices of ARVs, making it affordable for the government to provide AZT and other ARV combination therapies to ordinary South Africans.

The furore surrounding the Medicines Act of 1997 will be discussed in greater detail in the next chapter, but at this stage it is important to note that the government to some extent at least managed to provide some space for policy making unity between itself and members of the South African AIDS civil society. The latter were unified in their opposition to the pharmaceutical companies' court case against the South African government. However, it is significant that this unity was not sustainable nor sufficient to provide the solidarity and impetus required to put AIDS policy implementation back on a co-ordinated, cross-sectoral track. The government was as willing to use arguments of AZT's supposed toxicity when seeking to exculpate their own actions, or failure to act. The government's stance against the pharmaceutical companies did, however, succeed in garnering international support for its broader, anti-capitalist position, and this is widely credited for the loosening of IPRs regimes around ARVs that followed early in the new millennium.

Another important consequence of the government's AZT decision was the establishment of the Treatment Action Campaign (TAC) in December 1998. The TAC was founded by AIDS activists specifically to act as a watch-dog on the provision of treatment to PWAs (Ekambaram 1999: 11). Although this introduced an important player into the South African AIDS policy environment, it also led to an eventual further hardening of government versus civil society stances: in later years the TAC would use civil disobedience campaigns to create a critical mass against the ANC government's AIDS policies. Unfortunately, such a radicalisation of South Africa's AIDS civil society also translated into a crystallisation of government's focus on the value and strategy of prevention versus the broader AIDS civil society's insistence that treatment priorities were as important.[26] At the national political level, the party-political aspect of this drama came to the fore when the NP controlled Western Cape provincial government announced

26 The pro-treatment argument had been distilling for some years. Already in 1995 the Director of the Infectious Diseases Clinic at Johannesburg Hospital warned that '[w]e need an unambiguous commitment from the state regarding some form of antiretroviral therapy for our patients. However, patients, practitioners, pharmaceutical interest groups and the state need to co-operate together in the formulation of an acceptable treatment strategy. The silence of the current body politic in this regard is an ominous echo of a bygone era' (Spencer 1995: 34). Crewe (1996: 10) echoed this observation, noting that '[i]ronically the one key strategy on which almost no progress has been made is care and support – a strategy which can best be done by the [Department of Health] itself!'.

in early 1999 that they would, unilaterally and against the wishes of the central government, implement the rollout of MTCT programmes including the provision of AZT at certain public locations (Nattrass 2004: 49). This did not however end the drama around the government's AZT decision, which remained a feature up until the end of the Mandela administration in June 1999.

The third and shortest phase of public policy making during the Mandela administration commenced in October 1998, and came to an end with the swearing in of the first Mbeki Presidency in June 1999. What differentiates the few months between October 1998 and June 1999 is the announcement on 9 October 1998 of a new 'Partnership Against AIDS' by Deputy President Mbeki (Mbeki 1999: 576). In an effort to renew government's commitment against HIV and AIDS, the Mandela government had organised for the President himself to address the nation through a live television broadcast on 9 October, and to announce the latest iteration of the NAP: the 'Governmental AIDS Action Plan' (GAAP). AIDS activists were disappointed by the Deputy President's television performance – he was seen as wooden and cold towards the children surrounding him onscreen.

In addition to being a bit of a public relations disaster, Mbeki was at the last moment asked by Mandela to stand in for him – again AIDS activists took this as a sign that the Mandela government did not prioritise HIV and AIDS at the most senior governmental levels,[27] and the fact that Mbeki seemed unspontaneously wedded to the teleprompter led to criticism of the government simply going through the motions; lacking honesty. A month before the televised event the government held an AIDS crisis summit to launch the Partnership Against AIDS. However, the Minister of Health was late and Mbeki only made a brief appearance on the way to open a World Athletics meeting. Opposition parties suspected the partnership was a pre-election ploy (Van der Vliet 2001: 151).

The government had hoped that the limited level of co-operation with the South African AIDS civil society that came as a consequence of the government's popular resistance to pressure from pharmaceutical companies regarding the Medicines Act of 1997 would gather some momentum after the performance of October 1998. But the opposite happened: a mere two months later the TAC was established to a large part in response to the government's decision not to provide AZT to pregnant women.

The move to make AIDS notifiable

The short-lived ceasefire between the government and civil society dramatically came to an end in April 1999, when the government announced its intention to

27 As Van der Vliet (2001: 151) asked, 'Why did he fail the nation? Mandela had never made AIDS a priority, and his failure to participate in the program undermined the whole exercise. Why should the sceptical nation take AIDS seriously, when the President doesn't?'.

make HIV and AIDS a notifiable medical condition.[28] Again, this decision flew in the face of what had been agreed upon in earlier years. The NAP had been drafted as part of an evolving human rights-centred approach to AIDS, with the issue of patient confidentiality forming a central part of this culture. Significantly, the proposed notifiability measures were quite similar to ones that the NP government had introduced in 1987 – this was surprising, given the fact that the NP government was forced to withdraw the regulations a few years later. According to the Mandela government's proposed measures, medical practitioners would be required to report their findings to the local authorities or the Department of Health within 24 hours. Medical officers were to provide the age, sex, population group, date of diagnosis and any available information concerning the probable place and source of infection to the immediate family members and the persons who were giving care to the person in respect of whom the report is made (Van Wyk 1999: 3; ALQ 1999: 17–18).

This fourth 'scandal' did not come as a surprise to many AIDS policy observers: in November 1996 already the then Director General of Health, Dr Olive Shisana, expressed her unhappiness with the culture of 'secrecy' surrounding AIDS.[29] Shisana was at the time jeered by AIDS activists for comparing the danger of AIDS to the sensational and fast-killing Ebola virus. Again this was seen as government insensitivity towards PWAs and interpreted as wholly inappropriate, strengthening stigmatisation and driving the epidemic deeper underground (Karim 1999: 18). The NAP had been explicitly opposed to making AIDS a notifiable condition and at the time of its adoption government and civil society in South Africa were in agreement on this issue.

Furthermore, the Health Review of 1997 also warned against making AIDS notifiable and a dramatic illustration of existing prejudices in South Africa against PWAs was the murder in December 1998 of AIDS activist Gugu Dlamini, who was beaten to death by members of her community after she made her HIV status public (AIDS Analysis Africa 1999: 2). In addition to citing human rights concerns, experts cautioned the government against making AIDS notifiable in resource-constrained environments where there is limited access to health care and HIV testing and noted that notification is not an efficient way of collecting information on AIDS (Heywood 1999: 3; Smith 1999: 6; Colvin 1999: 4–5).

The fact that the government, in light of all these prior agreements, admonitions and events, was on 23 April 1999 still willing to gazette its unilateral intention to make AIDS notifiable mean't the wedge between itself and civil society was driven even deeper. The October 1998 armistice abruptly ended, and the AIDS civil society in South Africa declared open season on its own government. Government

28 Government Gazette R485, 23/4/99, Amendment to the Regulations Relating to Communicable Diseases and the Notification of Notifiable Medical Conditions.

29 Also, the Minister of Health in 1999 stated that it was time to treat AIDS as a public health issue and warned that 'the government would not be dictated to by NGOs and human rights activists' (Heywood 1999: 3).

countered – disastrously – by citing racism as being at the heart of such criticism. Also, Shisana's earlier position that opponents of making AIDS notifiable belonged to a Western, gay-centric subculture that did not fit into the South African context angered human rights activists (*Washington Post* 14 July 2000).[30] The AIDS Advisory Group (AAG) (originally set up by NP government in 1985) asked for a meeting with senior Health Department officials to clarify matters before the government's April 1999 statement, but the state responded by disbanding the body without any prior notice. Again this move angered AIDS activists outside of government; they accused the state of being unaccountable, undemocratic and intolerant of criticism.

High-ranking civil servants in the Ministry of Health routinely present themselves as being trapped between civil society and their impetuous political masters, and warn activists and medical practitioners not to 'offend' the politicians and to be 'constructive'. Whether intentional or not, the impression is created of a political leadership so concerned about status that it is prepared to act out of pique when criticised. This rather infantile approach to political debate and civil society mobilisation does not bode well for democracy or the rational resolution of AIDS policy debates (Nattrass 2004: 47).

This position echoed the Parliamentary Health Committee's earlier anxieties about the manner in which Minister Zuma was managing her portfolio (*Financial Mail* 14 June 1996):

> [i]n its report, the health committee lists several points of 'particular concern' about the department, raised in Parliamentary hearings and the media, which reinforce the Public Protector's portrait of a badly governed bureaucracy. The points include: transparency, accountability, adherence to public administration rules and regulations, sound preparation of new policies, development of a culture of consultation in policy development and proper reporting to Parliament.

The actual contents of these events are less important than the insights that they provide into the broader AIDS policy environment of the time. The manner in which the South African government and the AIDS civil society in particular related to them is quite instructive. For a start, the scandals were telling of the relationship between government and civil society. After the conceptualisation of the NAP in 1994 there were great hopes of the new democratic government and AIDS service organisations in civil society working together and co-ordinating their activities in order to combat the epidemic. By the end of the *Sarafina II* debacle, however, it was clear that a rift had been created between these two sets of policy agents – the idealism of the NACOSA process had all but dissolved.[31]

---

30 Taylor (1994: 9) noted that 'the AIDS lobby is seen…to be drawn from within the ranks of Gay Rights groups and liberal academics – frequently not talking the pragmatic bottom line…'.

31 Van der Vliet (2004b: 55) calls *Sarafina II* 'a watershed in relations between the Health Department and civil society. A NACOSA briefing to the Parliamentary portfolio

When reviewing the history of these scandals it again becomes clear how the politics of blame and the concomitant (re)politicisation of AIDS became an even stronger feature of the public policy environment in the second half of the 1990s. The blame cast on government's failure to implement the NAP, as well as the public sector and civil society's increasingly antagonistic and uncompromising positions can be seen as a feature of the fact that government was given and had taken on too much of the responsibility to 'save' South Africa from AIDS. The government became an easy scapegoat for those outside of the public sector and hence the state started to seek out scapegoats of its own. This forms an important context for our later discussion (Chapter 9) around possible reasons for government denial in responding to the epidemic.

---

committee on health (3 September 1996) states: "*Sarafina II* has done immense damage to the individuals and organizations active in the AIDS field. The process was not transparent and this has resulted in a rift between the Department of Health, NACOSA and the NGOs, as well as public derision and hostility to HIV and AIDS work and programmes"'.

Chapter 6
The Two Mbeki Governments' Responses to AIDS

A virus cannot cause a syndrome. A virus can cause a disease, and AIDS is not a disease, it is a syndrome.

Thabo Mbeki, 20 September 2000

Mbeki, Part 1: 1999–2004

In June 1999 Thabo Mbeki replaced Nelson Mandela as South African Head of State. The state-civil society relationship which had become strained after a series of AIDS 'scandals' after the mid-1990s remained so, thus failing to capitalise on the rapprochement around the government's legal case against large international pharmaceutical companies following on the enactment of the *Medicines and Related Substances Control Amendment Bill* (the 'Medicines Act') in 1997. But this was just one choppy wave of AIDS discontent that the new President's government would have to face in the years to come – in fact, Mbeki's governance of AIDS between 1999 and 2008 has six main features.

Firstly, the human rights culture nascent during the last years of the apartheid regime was entrenched during the Mandela period and could now be utilised to its fullest potential. After its establishment in the year before Mbeki took office, the Treatment Action Campaign (TAC) would now come to utilise the new national constitution and the legal environment that it created with the aim of ensuring People Living with HIV and AIDS's (PWAs) rights *vis-à-vis* essential drugs. For this reason the first theme of the Mbeki government's handling of HIV and AIDS would be the *culture of legislation and litigation* that came to accompany the governance of the South African AIDS epidemic. The significance of this culture for the role of the state in coping with AIDS became clear in the way in which civil society in particular increased its willingness to bypass the national government and go straight to the courts in order to achieve their goals, creating a kind of AIDS-governance-by-litigation.

The second important feature of the Mbeki government's management of AIDS is perhaps the most controversial, particularly in the manner in which it has been portrayed in the local and international media. Within four months of taking office Mbeki started to question the scientifically established causal link between the HI virus and AIDS, exacerbating the anti-intellectualism that also had been a characteristic of Mandela's AIDS governance. The President's so-called *denialism* and polemicisation of the science of AIDS (which started with the Virodene fiasco in 1997) further politicised and racialised the issue of AIDS in South African politics and at the policy level many observers would come to criticise the government for confusing the very conceptualisation of HIV and AIDS as a public policy problem, thus unduly and irresponsibly manipulating the policy agenda.

This crisis did not end during the first Mbeki government and it set into motion events that can be identified as the third main theme of the government's management of HIV and AIDS: its *handling of Mother-to-Child Transmission Prevention (MTCTP) and Highly Active Anti-Retroviral Therapy (HAART) programmes* in particular. The newly established human rights-oriented legal environment afforded civil society in South Africa with the opportunity to challenge the Mbeki government on its implementation of South Africans' constitutionally enshrined right to health. This legal environment, coupled with Mbeki's denialism, his practice of pseudo-science, and his continual questioning of AIDS statistics came to the fore in the shape of the TAC's ongoing battle to ensure the public availability of MTCT prevention programmes and ARVs in particular. Underpinning this struggle between the AIDS civil society and the South African government are varying positions on where fiscal priorities should lie (in zero sum terms): with either AIDS *prevention* programmes, or with AIDS *treatment*. Government took the former view, with the TAC and other members of the South African AIDS civil society emphasising the latter.

This issue provides a natural introduction to the fourth discernable theme of the Mbeki government's management of the South African AIDS epidemic: *the monetarisation of AIDS*. Increasingly AIDS pundits from both within the government and civil society began to emphasise the financial costs of AIDS – both in terms of costs to the South African society and economy, as well as the costs associated with an appropriate publicly funded response. Importantly, the public monetarisation of AIDS in South Africa really commenced in the mid-1990s, when the Mandela government enacted legislation to force large pharmaceutical companies to make ARVs available in this country as well as in the rest of the developing world.

The fifth theme of Mbeki's AIDS management was the ongoing attempt to reappraise the structural variables that drive the epidemic in this country. Since AIDS first emerged in South Africa, the morality and ethics of the state's response has been under the microscope. The thematic golden thread that runs through all the rhetoric surrounding this epidemic points in a single direction: *unequal gender relations, culture and race*. What does the history of dealing with HIV and AIDS tell one about South African society? How has the South African government's conceptualisation of who is to blame, of who the enemy is and how one should respond as a society had an impact on the state's capacity to respond?

The sixth and final theme of Mbeki's management of the epidemic refers to the government's 'AIDS rehabilitation' between August 2006 and September 2008. In the two years preceding Thabo Mbeki's dramatic departure from government there was an ostensible realignment of the National Department of Health's and civil society's relationship regarding the future management of AIDS in South Africa. The 16th Global AIDS Conference held in Toronto in August 2006 was critical in presaging this development since it made the government's final loss of the moral high ground at the domestic as well as international AIDS environments painfully explicit. Also, demonstrable recent spikes in South African AIDS mortality levels had rendered any denial of the growing impact of the epidemic ridiculous. The imperative for a radical change in the manner in which AIDS had been managed until the second half of 2006 was also made clear by advances in medical technologies, as well as by their increasing affordability. These factors along with the South African Minister of Health's temporary departure from the political scene created an environment in which pragmatism could prevail. The result was a more focused rapprochement between government and civil society groups, which in turn resulted in the successful drafting (and publication, in March 2007) of an inclusive and legitimate *HIV and AIDS and STI Strategic Plan for South Africa: 2007–2011.*

That Mbeki's tenure was fraught with instances of denialism (as the contestation of mainstream AIDS science) is certainly not unknown. However, the extent to which denial as a whole was an element in government's response at that time has been explored to a much lesser extent. Applying Cohen's wider definition of official denial (as set out in Chapter 3) to the Mbeki era thus allows us to look beyond the much debated instances of AIDS denialism and to explore other ways in which the issue could have been sidelined or denied. This puts Mbeki's legacy of inaction on a much more even keel to his predecessors' responses and therefore facilitates a more balanced assessment of the history of official rhetoric that has shaped South Africa's response to the epidemic. Moreover, looking beyond the instances of AIDS denialism, allows us to bolster our initial proposition that denial is likely to have been a motivator of government's actions long before Mbeki's rule.

The institutional and legal context

The HIV and AIDS and STD Strategic Plan for South Africa: 2000–05

Within the first month of Mbeki's Presidential inauguration in June 1999 the institutional wheels were set in motion for the creation of the new government's key policy document on HIV and AIDS. At a planning meeting held early in July 1999 the government decided that the National AIDS Plan (NAP) of 1994 should be 'revisited and revised' (Crewe 1999: 31) – not, it is important to note, abandoned altogether, but amended in accordance with the AIDS policy challenges facing the new government. The Mbeki government realised that it would not be necessary to scrap the NAP of 1994 – after all, that policy document had the buy-in of all the main AIDS policy actors both in- and outside of government and it was widely lauded as an ideal policy for South Africa. Hence, at the meeting it was agreed that a committee would be appointed and charged with the development of a five-year HIV and AIDS and STD Strategic Plan. Task teams were established to review existing goals and objectives for the designated priority areas and after follow-up meetings in September and October 1999 a draft document was presented to the Inter-Ministerial Committee in November (with additional comments solicited from all government Ministers). The final document – the 'HIV and AIDS and STDs Strategic Plan for South Africa: 2000–2005' – was completed in January 2000.

The Strategic Plan of 2000 (see Table 6.1) stated that all government departments, organisations and stakeholders would use the document as the basis to develop their own strategic and operational plans so that all the initiatives for the country as a whole could be harmonised to maximise effectiveness and efficiency.

Table 6.1 Outline of the HIV and AIDS and STD Strategic Plan for South Africa: 2000–05

The primary goals: Reduce the number of new HIV infections (especially among youth) Reduce the impact of HIV and AIDS on individuals, families and communities
Four main areas:
1. Prevention Goal 1: Promote safe and healthy sexual behaviour Goal 2: Improve the management and control of STDs Goal 3: Reduce mother to child transmission Goal 4: Address issues relating to blood transfusion and HIV Goal 5: Provide appropriate post-exposure services Goal 6: Improve access to voluntary HIV testing and counselling
2. Treatment, care and support Goal 7: Provide treatment, care and support services in health facilities Goal 8: Provide adequate treatment, care and support services in the community Goal 9: Develop and expand the provision of care to children and orphans
3. Monitoring, research and surveillance Goal 10: Ensure AIDS vaccine development Goal 11: Investigate treatment and care options Goal 12: Conduct policy research Goal 13: Conduct regular surveillance
4. Human and legal rights Goal 14: Create an appropriate social environment Goal 15: Develop an appropriate legal and policy environment

Source: Adapted from Smart (2002:193) and the Strategic Plan (2000).

It was the aim of the Plan for every government ministry and every sector to have dedicated HIV and AIDS focal persons. In addition to reaffirming the majority of the key principles and programmatic imperatives referred to in the NAP of 1994 (and in the National Health Review of 1997), the Strategic Plan of 2000 also made specific reference to a number of institutional structures that would drive the programme's implementation during the Mbeki administration. These structures included the creation of a South African National AIDS Council (SANAC), the interdepartmental committee on AIDS (IDC), the Health Ministers of each of the nine provinces (MinMECs), a committee consisting of all provincial heads of health (the Provincial Health Restructuring Committee (PHRC)), provincial AIDS councils (PACs), a Directors General forum, as well as a reconfirmation of the central role of the Department of Health's HIV and AIDS and STD Directorate.

The content of the Strategic Plan of 2000 was praised for its holistic view and comprehensive grasp of the issues that needed to be addressed in order for South Africa to prevail in the battle against AIDS. However, the breakdown between the (ideal) programmatic prescriptions and institutional structures of the Plan on the one hand and the implementation of those strategies on the other hand very soon became all too apparent. The Plan appeared to be unable to overcome successive ANC governments' crises of implementation, of moving from policy conceptualisation to operationalisation. We discuss the policy environment that curtailed the successful implementation of the Strategic Plan of 2000 in greater detail below, but at this stage it is worth examining some of the criticisms levelled against the actual plan.

Reviewing priority area four of the Strategic Plan of 2000 two years after it was made public, Mark Heywood (2002: 2) noted that 'the inertia and invisibility of the SANAC for the most of 2001 prevented [the devising of implementation strategies] from taking place'. Expressing frustration with the fact that, although South Africa had developed one of the most progressive and far-sighted policy and legislative environments relating to HIV of any country in the world, Heywood (2002: 3) continued to say that 'the policy environment has still not catalysed implementation'. The government's decision to oppose the decriminalisation of commercial sex work as well as its reticence to roll out ARV therapies and MTCT prevention programmes at public facilities (a problem which continued up until the very end of the Mbeki administration) was also taken to indicate unwillingness on the part of the state to act on the prescriptions of its own Strategic Plan.

This poses an interesting question: in drawing up an AIDS policy framework that says one thing, but then explicitly failing to act on it, what was the Mbeki government's true policy on HIV and AIDS? As will be noted below, this question became a refrain throughout the entire Mbeki administration – the main point at this stage is to note that there appeared to be a disquieting inability (some would say unwillingness) on the part of the South African government to effectively implement all the prescriptions of the Strategic Plan. On this basis, government's implementation of the Strategic Plan is raised again in later discussions of Cohen's classification of official denial, as another possible case of partial acknowledgement (Chapter 8).

Further illustrating this point, Hickey et al. (2003: 11) note that the Strategic Plan of 2000 was 'criticised for lacking a clear commitment to treatment options, such as the provision of ARV therapy, as well as lacking clear and measurable plans, timeframes and a dedicated budget for implementation'. They also point to a fault line inherent to the Plan specific to difficulties at the interface between national and provincial policy implementation:

- The provinces – without being provided with adequate resources – have tended to be primarily responsible for the implementation of policy.
- Provincial programmes lacked an independent evaluation system; and
- There appeared to have been little inter-provincial collaboration or communication (Hickey et al. 2003: 13).

The official provincial government AIDS response, created in November 1999 and entitled the 'National Integrated Plan' (NIP) further illustrates these challenges. The NIP focused on the Life Skills programme in primary and secondary schools, the voluntary counselling and testing (VCT) programme, and the community and home-based care and support (CHBC) programme, and was jointly delivered by the health, education and welfare sectors (government's so-called Social Cluster) and was funded separately from the regular budget process. However, Hickey (2001: 1) as well as Agenda (2002: 96) found that the NIP struggled to implement and co-ordinate broad policy objectives, decision making in HIV and AIDS budget allocations, had cumbersome administrative structures and struggled to develop the capacity for effective implementation. An illustration of this is the fact that 'in the first year of the NIP, the provinces managed to spend only 36.5 per cent of the total HIV and AIDS grants available to them from the central government' (SAPA 14 November 2001).

Some of the most strident criticism against the Strategic Plan of 2000 was centred on the particulars surrounding the creation in January 2000 of SANAC. In terms of the Plan, SANAC was the natural product of the government's stated commitment to an inter-sectoral approach to AIDS. 'Furthermore', Strode and Grant (2004: 14) write, 'SANAC had to replace the AIDS Advisory Council, as it was not a multi-sectoral body and only made up of technical experts'. The Strategic Plan of 2000 described the role of SANAC as:

- Advising the government on HIV and AIDS policy.
- Advocating for the effective involvement of sectors and organisations in implementing programmes and strategies.
- Monitoring the implementation of the Strategic Plan in all sectors of society.
- Creating and strengthening partnerships for an expanded response amongst all sectors.
- Mobilising resources for the implementation of AIDS programmes; and
- Recommending appropriate research.

The Strategic Plan of 2000 also provided that SANAC was to be made up of 34 people, 16 from government and 17 from various sectors of civil society. It further provided that SANAC should be chaired by the Deputy President of South Africa. Once again, on paper the creation of SANAC could not be faulted: it could potentially provide a vessel which could heal the wounds and animosity created by the *Sarafina II* and other AIDS scandals during the Mandela administration; it could be an effective interface between central government (via the presence and chairmanship of the Deputy President) and AIDS civil society in South Africa, providing the institutional vector for the efficient implementation of the programmatic features of the Strategic Plan. The reality, however, turned out much different. Within weeks of its launch SANAC became the target of a barrage of criticism from both the South African media and the vast majority of members of the country's AIDS civil society: its membership was unilaterally appointed by the government, the majority of SANAC members were government officials, there was an all but total absence of scientists, clinicians and pharmaceutical company representatives and the AIDS Consortium (a network representing about 200 NGOs) were wholly excluded from its composition (Galloway 2000: 15). As Trengove-Jones (2001: 31) noted:

> [t]hrougout 2000 we saw mounting tensions within what could only ironically be termed a 'partnership' against AIDS. Designed in part to give new urgency and impetus to the partnership, [SANAC] was launched early in the new year, top heavy with government Ministers and lacking almost any significant NGO representation. The rift this caused only widened through the year until the gap between the government and NGOs had grown to the point where, in October, the AIDS Law Project and the TAC gave notice of their intention to take the government to court over its refusal to implement programmes for MTCT prophylaxis.

In an independent review of the SANAC, Strode and Grant (2004: 24–36) found that:

- It has proved to be ineffective in advising the government on any matters of great policy significance.
- Its structure does not allow it to monitor the implementation.
- Its structure does not allow it to interact with other stakeholders or any non-members.
- Its structure has not enabled it to form strategic partnerships with other organisations.
- Its meetings are closed (making it all but impossible to hold SANAC accountable through the normal democratic channels).
- It is for all intents and purposes managed by the Department of Health.
- It is unable to make an impact on the outcome of key decisions that are made.

- It has no capacity to monitor the implementation of the Strategic Plan; and
- It is not bringing political commitment to the HIV and AIDS response in South Africa.

Criticism against SANAC thus centred on the fact that it was not representative of the South African AIDS community, as had been envisaged in the Strategic Plan of 2000. On the contrary, it was viewed as an exclusive, government-heavy institution created to rubber-stamp and legitimise the national Department of Health's questionable response to the AIDS epidemic. Many members of South Africa's non-governmental AIDS elite were calling for the scrapping or radical reconstitution of SANAC. Similarly, problems remained that kept the IDC from carrying out its mandate. These included insufficient links between the IDC and the Directors General social cluster, the junior position of most IDC members, lack of communication between IDC members and their senior management, insufficient resources allocated to HIV and AIDS programmes within departments and insufficient project management and monitoring in many departments. Also, due to a high turnover in staff, skills building is an ongoing need; there was a lack in programme management skills.

Legislation and case law

Legislation had been used by the National Party government before the end of apartheid in an attempt to compensate for a lack of AIDS-specific programmatic policy initiatives. This situation changed under the Mandela government, where the National AIDS Coordinating Committee of South Africa (NACOSA) process had led to the drafting of the NAP of 1994. Legislation then became a complementary tool in the state's arsenal in the fight against HIV and AIDS, particularly in so far as it reflected the establishment of South Africa's culture of human rights. As Forman et al. (2003: 13) noted:

> [l]egislation plays a critical role in achieving health reform goals, and has a multidirectional and dialogic relationship with policy. On the one hand, legislation depends on the development of policy to guide its nature and content. Yet health legislation can also express and formulate health policies, and through statutes and regulations it can shape the way that health policy is translated into health programmes and services. Legislation however plays a distinct role from policy, and serves to coordinate health sector activities, and to create a management and administrative framework for the development of health care systems. It establishes structures and mechanisms to put policy into practice and provides for sanctions should the policy (encapsulated in the legal provisions) be breached. Health legislation creates certainty with respect to what is expected from various role-players and what the user of health services can expect.

In particular, legislation was used to regulate the workplace and to create a fair and non-discriminatory environment for individuals to apply for and retain employment. Echoing the human rights principles set out in the Constitution of 1996, the *Labour Relations Act*, *Basic Conditions of Employment Act* and the *Employment Equity Act* were but three pieces of legislation introduced during the Mandela administration that contained specific measures to safeguard the rights of HIV-positive individuals. The human rights approach of such formal legislation was also reflected in the Case Law that was evolving: focusing on the world of work, several cases came before the courts that further entrenched the rights of PWAs and a powerful legal foundation was established for the protection of patient-doctor confidentiality, as well as the protection of the rights of HIV-positive employees and job applicants. Litigation was actually becoming an increasingly important strategy in civil society's as well as individuals' efforts to force the government to stop prevaricating on the provision of MTCT prevention and ARV therapies.

During the first Mbeki administration several important pieces of legislation as well as Case Law came to fruition or were introduced which further served to entrench a human rights approach to HIV and AIDS. The *Medicines Act* of 1997 was the first and had the highest media profile – both domestically and internationally. In brief, the Act contained provisions that would make it possible for the South African government to parallel import ARVs from abroad and to issue compulsory licenses to local pharmaceutical manufacturers to produce generic AIDS drugs at a fraction of what it would cost to purchase such drugs from their foreign patent holders. Such measures are legal under the WTO TRIPS rules (of which South Africa is a signatory), but the *Medicines Act* became controversial when the US-based Pharmaceutical Manufacturers' Association (PhrMA) (representing 39 pharmaceutical companies) decided in 1998 to take the Mandela government to court on this issue. During the second half of the Mandela administration the American government placed immense pressure on the South Africans to honour the patent rights of the American companies who developed the drugs, going so far as to put South Africa on the US 'Super 301' trade watch list. Many observers accused the American government of using bullying tactics in an effort to put profits above the rights of PWAs and eventually the issue became a political and public relations disaster for the American government.

The South African government (both under Mandela and in the early years of the Mbeki administration) did manage, however, to put the issue of PWAs' rights to essential drugs on the international agenda. The issue also garnered wide support from sectors of civil society; the TAC and the trade union COSATU in particular established links to drive popular resistance and demonstrations against the PhrMA court action. In April 2001 the PhrMA decided to withdraw their case against the South African government and this caused great elation amongst South African and international AIDS communities, who hailed this move as a victory for human rights in the context of HIV and AIDS. The South African government had triumphed in a David vs. Goliath battle against big business. However, the elation was short-lived: at the news conference following the PhrMA's decision to withdraw their legal challenge, the South African Minister of Health (Dr Manto Tshabalala-Msimang) announced that the drugs remained too expensive to parallel import, or to manufacture locally.

This startling flip-flop in government rhetoric qualifies it as a likely instance of implicatory official denial. The Health Minister's apparent unwillingness to embrace the now radically discounted treatment suggested that government's initial arguments that pharmaceutical patents were hampering South Africa's AIDS response could have simply been a diversionary smoke screen. As we argue in Chapter 7, by blaming pharmaceutical giants for the extent of the epidemic, the government could construct itself as a victim and in so doing absolved itself from accountability. Whilst government's challenging of patents is essentially entirely just, and as was reflected by civil society's support for this action, righteous and proactive, it is their sudden change in position on this issue that cast doubt on their motive.

The alliance between government and the South African AIDS civil society came to a bitter end, with the latter accusing the government of not being willing to follow through on their promises to make these drugs available to PWAs. 'To date, little has come of this victory, a failure which, as a *Business Day* editorial at the time suggested, would leave "the impression that government is more interested in scoring points off the multinationals than providing care for millions of poor HIV and AIDS sufferers"' (Van der Vliet 2004: 63).

This introduced a phase of severe conflict between particularly the TAC and the South African government, as will be discussed in greater detail below.

However, the drama surrounding the *Medicines Act* of 1997 did serve a number of purposes:

- The Government succeeded in putting the issue of patients' access to essential drugs on the global policy agenda and in doing so aligned itself with global human rights and AIDS activists.
- The PhrMAs' retreat was seen as a moral and legal victory for PWAs, further entrenching a human rights-centric approach to drugs provision (particularly in the developing world).
- It paved the way for the South African and other developing country governments to declare AIDS a health emergency and to activate the TRIPS provisions that would ensure legal parallel importation and generic manufacturing of AIDS drugs (Kasper 2002: 157).
- However, the South African government's bizarre about-turn on applying the Act served to drive the wedge between civil society and the state very deep. The government's explanation of fiscal constraints was viewed as an unjustified cop-out. In Buch's (2004: 95) analysis, 'having led the world with its challenge, South Africa announced that it would not be implementing what it had fought for. This made the victory somewhat hollow…*Government's AIDS policy is solid, but its actions and signals have been mixed*' [italics added].

In addition to the conclusion in 2001 of the commotion surrounding the *Medicines Act* of 1998 there were three other developments in AIDS-specific legislation that were significant during the first Mbeki administration. In the first place, in August 1999 Chapter II of the *Employment Equity Act* (EEA) 55 of 1998 came into effect. Chapter II is specifically aimed at eradicating unfair discrimination in the workplace. Amongst other measures, the EEA prohibits any person from unfairly discriminating against an employee on grounds of their HIV status. Furthermore, medical testing prior to employment is outlawed, and the Act makes a point of listing HIV status as a ground separate from the ground of disability. According to Du Plessis (2000: 3) 'the EEA is the first piece of legislation in the world that offers protection specifically to persons living with HIV from unfair discrimination and unauthorised HIV testing'. However, there was some criticism against the more recent versions of the Act, which do not go far enough in expressly prohibiting insurance companies from discriminating against PWAs (ALQ 1999: 4) – such criticisms have led some legal experts to note that a review of the EEA might be in order (Joni and Heywood 2001: 11).

Secondly, in 2001 the South African Law Commission drafted a Bill for the Minister of Justice that provides for court-ordered compulsory HIV testing of persons arrested in sexual offence cases. The draft Bill presented the government with a legal conundrum: under South Africa's legal constitution, one is innocent until proven guilty – also in cases of sexual assault or rape. However, the draft legislation would force someone merely accused of a sexual offence to undergo a medical test to ascertain HIV status (Goyer 2001: 8).

Thirdly, in January 2001 the government retreated on its intention (gazetted in the first half of 1999) to make AIDS a notifiable medical condition. In their explanation for this move, the Department of Health cited the burden of stigma that this might exacerbate as its main consideration. The government also noted that they did not have the infrastructure in place to enforce any notifiability regulation or legislation (SAPA 4 April 2001). This change of heart on the part of the government was a victory for human rights activists, who noted that measures or legislation to make AIDS notifiable would have clashed with human rights standards: '[t]he regulations would have required non-consensual disclosure of AIDS status to a broad range of health care workers, as well as to immediate family member and caregivers' (Forman et al. 2003: 19).

Besides these developments in the legislative context, the first Mbeki administration also saw some advances in the terrain of Case Law affecting HIV and AIDS. As noted earlier, the TAC and the AIDS Law Project in particular set an important precedent during the first Mbeki administration in using Case Law to force the state to provide MTCT prevention and ARV therapies at public facilities. Two instances of the use of Case Law regarding HIV and AIDS merit further mention.

Interestingly, both cases dealt with applicants for work at South African Airways (SAA). These cases were first brought before the South African courts during the Mandela administration, but concluded during the Mbeki administration. In the first of these, *Hoffman v SAA*, the applicant in 1998 contended that SAA had unfairly discriminated against him on the basis of his HIV-positive status in rejecting his application for employment as a flight attendant. In 2001 the court ruled in favour of the applicant, noting that the SAA's employment policy was in contravention of the applicant's right to equity. In September 2000 the Constitutional Court upheld Hoffman's application, 'alter[ing] the legal landscape concerning AIDS in the workplace in Southern Africa' (Motebele and Heywood 2001: 10).

In the second case, *'A' v SAA*, the applicant had also been refused employment by the SAA on the basis of his HIV status. The case was one of the first such cases to be heard in the Labour Court, and the SAA's pre-employment HIV testing policy was successfully challenged. 'A' was awarded R100,000 as compensation, with SAA unconditionally admitting that the exclusion of 'A' from the position of cabin attendant on the grounds of his HIV status was unjustified (Figueira 2000: 12). Both of these cases have set important precedents in the South African legal system as well as in the HIV and AIDS policy environment, enforcing the human rights of job applicants, as well as the measures set out in the EEA.

Denialism and obfuscation: Mbeki enters the fray

According to Barnett and Whiteside (2002: 335) political leadership is a necessary but not sufficient criterion for preventing the spread of HIV or turning the epidemic round. This must begin at the highest levels if there is to be national success. However, South Africa provides an example where the absence of clear and decisive leadership damaged prevention efforts.

Political leadership refers to proactive and effective action from the top echelons of government to drive the battle against the epidemic. This includes the Head of State as well as key government functionaries and departments. There seems to be a prevailing judgment amongst AIDS commentators that as far as AIDS is concerned Thabo Mbeki did more harm than good after assuming power in 1999. This reputation became established even when Mbeki was still Mandela's Deputy: his first foray into the AIDS arena came in 1997 when he supported Virodene as an alleged cure for AIDS. Despite scientific evidence to the contrary Mbeki pushed for the registration of the drug and when the MCC refused to do so, this medical peer review body was first excoriated as being racist or 'counter-transformationalist' and then later on unceremoniously disbanded and politically reconstituted. Mbeki never distanced himself from Virodene or corrected his previous stance and drove the wedge between mainstream AIDS science in South Africa and the government even deeper when, a year or so later, he questioned the efficacy of AZT – yet again making statements that flew in the face of established medical science, as well as scientific evidence. As a consequence, the Mandela government refused to provide AZT for women who had been raped.

Mbeki's 'discovery' that AZT might have negative side-effects was gleaned during Internet searches and Crewe (2000: 123) believes that these debates around the safety of ARVs led him to the so-called dissident views on the causal link between HIV and AIDS. As discussed in detail in Chapter 3, dissidents are a small and diverse minority group of scientists and other individuals, some of whom do not believe that HIV causes AIDS, others who believe that HIV does not exist at all and a third group who believe that HIV is the cause of AIDS but that it is all a plot by the pharmaceutical companies to sell drugs. These dissidents' views on the existence and causal links between HIV and AIDS have been repeatedly refuted in the 1980s and 1990s by clear scientific evidence that the HI virus exists, that it has been isolated (and in fact photographed) and that it leads to immunosuppression and eventually the physio-pathological syndrome called AIDS.

However, the Virodene and AZT sagas during the Mandela administration created a policy environment around HIV and AIDS which manifested in a hugely defensive and obdurate government – not in all cases reflecting the views of technocrats and lesser functionaries, but certainly views of some of the political elite within the state. Instead of establishing a culture of free and open exchange between the government and AIDS civil society in South Africa, this served to entrench a growing mistrust and eventual disgust and overt antagonism (even several instances of litigation) between these two groups that are so critical for the fight against the epidemic. Eventually, these fault lines manifested within the governing alliance (ANC-SACP-COSATU) itself, with the latter two members of that alliance censuring the ANC government for aligning itself with discredited views beyond the fringes of mainstream science.

A brief chronology of Mbeki's assault on AIDS orthodoxy reads as follows:

1999:

- In late October in a speech before the National Council of Provinces (NCOP) Mbeki refers to the alleged toxicity of AZT and requests his new Minister of Health to undertake further investigations about its safety and efficacy.
- The ANC's annual report notes that AZT would not be made available at public facilities.

2000:

- Early in the year the impending formation of a Presidential AIDS Panel is announced. The panel includes mainstream as well as dissident scientists in an effort to explore opposing viewpoints on the causal link between HIV and AIDS. From then onwards official AIDS discourses on this causation refers to the causal link between HIV and AIDS as a 'thesis'.
- In February Mbeki questions the orthodox aetiology of AIDS, earning a rebuke from the chairperson of the South African Medical Association (SAMA), which represents 17,000 South African doctors (including 75 per cent of all doctors in active practice in both the private and public sectors). Mbeki also rebukes the head of the MRC, Professor Malegapuru Makgoba, for failing to read a particular article about the toxicity of AZT.

- In April, Mbeki tells the ANC's Parliamentary caucus that drug companies are financing the TAC, which was now 'infiltrating' the trade unions.
- In March, the Presidential spokesman, Parks Mankahlana, accuses a large pharmaceutical company of being 'like the marauders of the military industrial complex who propagated fear to increase their profits' (Lodge 2002: 257).
- In April, Mbeki writes a letter to world leaders (including Tony Blair and Bill Clinton) in which he hails AIDS dissidents as modern-day Galileos. The White House finds the letter so bizarre that at first it doubts its authenticity. There appear to be cracks within the ruling ANC on this issue, with the MEC for health in Kwa-Zulu Natal attacking AIDS dissidents for abusing their access to the President to spread lies and confusion.
- Between June and October the President and the leader of the official opposition, Tony Leon, exchange letters on the subject of AIDS. Mbeki reiterates his doubts about the efficacy and safety of ARVs. In subsequent letters to Leon, Mbeki refers to 'hysterical' estimates of the incidence of AIDS by epidemiologists and the 'insulting' theory that AIDS originated in Africa.
- In June 2000, the President opens the 13th International AIDS Conference in Durban, reiterates his doubts about the South African epidemic and states that poverty (and not HIV) is the main contributing factor to AIDS. Earlier, in response to journalist Charlene Smith's public appeal that South Africans exercise some cultural introspection about the high incidence of rape and sexual assault in the country, Mbeki accuses Smith of launching a blatant racist attack on the new South Africa. Five thousand scientists sign the Durban Declaration, reiterating the mainstream scientific view regarding HIV and AIDS, but the President's spokesman later notes that the declaration is fit for the dustbin, and that it is an 'elitist' document.
- In September, in an interview with *Time Magazine*, Mbeki casts doubts on whether HIV (if it exists) is the only contributing factor to AIDS. Later in the month, in a statement to Parliament, Mbeki states that a virus (HIV) cannot cause a syndrome (AIDS) – echoing the statements of dissidents. After his statement to Parliament, the SACP and COSATU call on Mbeki to stop raising questions about the causes of AIDS in public. The ANC health portfolio committee in Parliament sends a confidential memorandum to the Minister of Health urging her and Mbeki to make a public statement stating that HIV causes AIDS (Sparks 2003: 295). After an ANC National Executive Council (NEC) meeting later on in the month, Mbeki announces that he would make no further public statements on the issue. Behind closed doors, however, Mbeki continues his crusade; if newspaper reports are to be believed (*Mail & Guardian*, 28 September 2000), in late September he addresses the ANC's Parliamentary caucus, stating that the American intelligence agency (the CIA) and large drug companies were behind a conspiracy to discredit him. Mbeki allegedly also accuses the TAC of being

funded by these drug companies and that they were leading the local assault against his presidency. He also states that it was not clear to him whether his own Cabinet supported him against the drug companies.

- In early October, the ANC's NEC publishes a statement stating that Mbeki was the target of a massive onslaught against the ANC and the government. The statement criticises the SACP and COSATU for supporting views counter to those held by Mbeki. However, the statement also announces that government policy on AIDS would continue on the 'premise' that HIV causes AIDS. The AIDS issue is taken up in electioneering in the Western Cape. Responding to the opposition's undertaking to supply free ARVs in the province, Mbeki notes that South Africans were being used as 'guinea pigs' and the provincial government's prescription of such dangerous medication could be compared to the biological warfare of the apartheid era (*Mail & Guardian*, 26 October 2000).

2001:

- In an address to Parliament in March, Mbeki defends his decision not to declare AIDS a national emergency, saying that '[n]o other country has declared a state of emergency on these grounds' (*Washington Post*, 15 March 2001).
- In April the Presidential AIDS Panel reports. Its members fail to find consensus either about the causes of AIDS or as to how the epidemic should be contained. Two parallel sets of recommendations are presented, reflecting the division between mainstream and dissident science. (Four years later, after she had left government, the former head of the government's AIDS Directorate, Dr Nono Simelela, noted that:

  > I sat at these meetings and I listened to these international scientists failing to agree on anything…The dialogue became pathetic. They were swearing at each other on email; they were calling each other names. Some of the emails we had to mediate were scary' (Gill 2006: 63).

  In later media interviews, Mbeki remains adamant that a virus cannot cause a syndrome, and he publicly refuses to take an HIV test, stating that such an act would reflect an embrace on his part of the mainstream view that HIV causes AIDS.
- In an August interview, Mbeki casts doubt on the accuracy of statistics demonstrating that AIDS has become the main killer of adult South Africans. He tells the BBC that crime is the main killer in the country. In the same month Mbeki requests his Minister of Health to reassess the government's policy on AIDS, citing seven-year-old WHO statistics noting that AIDS is a comparatively minor cause of death in South Africa. In a letter to Tshabalala-Msimang, Mbeki states that:

> [n]eedless to say these figures will provoke a howl of displeasure and a concerted propaganda campaign among those who have convinced themselves that HIV and AIDS is the single biggest cause of death in our country. These are the people whose prejudices led them to discover the false reality, among other things, that we are running out of space in our cemeteries as a result of unprecedented deaths caused by HIV and AIDS… Nevertheless, whatever the intensity of the hostile propaganda that might be provoked by the WHO statistics, we cannot allow that government policy and programmes should be informed by misperceptions, however widespread and well established they may seem to be…(*Business Day* 10 September 2001).

- In October leaks from an MRC report suggests that the WHO statistics are ridiculously outdated and that AIDS is, indeed, the main cause of adult mortality in South Africa. The office of the President delays the publication of the MRC report, calling its findings 'not credible'. In a speech at the University of Fort Hare, Mbeki launches a vociferous attack on AIDS activists and the medical establishment, saying that:

> others who consider themselves to be our leaders take to the streets carrying their placards to demand that because [black people] are germ carriers and human beings of a lower order that cannot subject their passions to reason, we must perforce adopt strange opinions to save a depraved and diseased people from perishing from a self-inflicted disease (Mbeki 2001).

- In November the Parliamentary Joint Standing Committee on the Improvement of the Quality of Life and Status of Women (a committee dominated by ANC women members) releases a report countering the President's position, requesting the immediate provision of ARVs to rape survivors and to prevent MTCT. Subsequently the TAC takes the government to court in an effort to force the state to make such provisions. When the court rules in favour of the TAC, the Minister of Health decides to appeal to the Constitutional Court on the grounds that it was not within the authority of the courts to make health policy. Early in 2002 the Court rejects the government's application.

2002:

- Early in the year the government faces increasing opposition to its stance on the provision of ARVs, with Mandela, Archbishop Desmond Tutu, the ANC's Gauteng premier, COSATU, the SACP and the Anglican Church calling for the speedy rollout of ARV programmes. The ANC's spokesman, Smuts Ngonyama, issues a statement criticising the visiting former US President Jimmy Carter for a similar call on the government.

- In March the ANC NEC announces that an ARV rollout programme would only follow on a study to determine the drugs' safety and efficacy and that such a study would only be concluded towards the end of the year.
- News breaks of an extraordinary document entitled 'Castro Hlongwane, Caravans, Cats, Geese, Foot and Mouth, and Statistics: HIV and AIDS and the Struggle for the Humanisation of the African' that circulates among ANC NEC members. The document reiterates dissident rhetoric and again points to a conspiracy between the media and scientists to sell the idea of an African AIDS epidemic, largely in favour of the consumption of ARVs. It attacks 'Eurocentric science' and 'mental colonisation' and insists that Africa must reject the idea that is a victim of a self-inflicted disease called AIDS.[1]
- After its legal defeat, in April the government announces that ARVs would, in fact, be rolled out at public facilities, but again rollout is delayed – to such an extent that the TAC again takes legal action in December to force the Mpumalanga provincial government to start rolling out ARVs. The National Minister of Health states that, were the province's MEC for health to go to prison, 'I'm going with her' (Van der Vliet 2004: 75).
- At the Barcelona Global AIDS conference in June, Tshabalala-Msimang responds to the earlier Constitutional Court ruling, saying that the government 'will implement because we are forced to implement…I must give my people poison' (Van der Vliet 2004: 76).
- In September NEDLAC announces a task team to negotiate a plan for the rollout of ARVs. The TAC and COSATU are partners at the negotiating table. However, the government announces that it will refuse to sign the agreement, leading to a civil disobedience campaign by the TAC.
- Mbeki barely mentions AIDS at the ANC party congress in December.

2003:

- Mbeki's state of the nation address at the opening of Parliament in February devotes only two sentences, in a 21-page speech, to AIDS.
- In March the Health Minister advocates that PWAs take garlic and olive oil rather than 'toxic' ARVs to boost their immune systems. Mbeki does not make any public statement on the furore that follows this statement, leading Van der Vliet (2004: 77) to ask:

> How does a Minister with such a string of gaffes and blunders behind her – and the strong suspicion that she herself is an AIDS 'denialist' – retain her portfolio?…If she is not censured, disciplined or fired for her sayings

1 Six years later, Mark Gevisser, Thabo Mbeki's biographer, revealed that Mbeki himself was the author of this document. Gevisser stated that '[t]here is no question as to the message Thabo Mbeki was delivering to me along with this document: he was now, as he had been since 1999, an AIDS dissident' (*The Guardian*, 6 November 2007).

> and doings, there is a simple explanation. It's because Thabo Mbeki wants it that way. However low a profile Mbeki keeps on the AIDS issue these days, nothing he has done refutes [this].

- Also in March, American journalist Samantha Power (2003: 67) reports on a conversation between Mbeki and a prominent Cabinet member:

> 'I've been to so many AIDS funerals', the Minister said. 'I attend more every month'.
>
> The President was irritated by the comment. 'What makes you so sure they died of AIDS?'
>
> The official explained that young men in their twenties and thirties don't just die of pneumonia.
>
> 'Yes', Mbeki said, 'but you don't really know how they died, do you?'

- In response to the TAC's civil disobedience campaign (which enjoys wide support from COSATU) the Minister of Health in April launches a scathing attack on the bona fides of TAC leadership, accusing them of racism. Tshabalala-Msimang also attacks the KwaZulu-Natal province for having submitted (and won) an application to the Global Fund in Geneva for US$72 million, aimed at ARV rollout.
- In an interview in July with the BBC, Mbeki again questions statistics demonstrating that hundreds of South Africans die every day due to AIDS.
- In an interview with the *Washington Post* in September, Mbeki denies having known anyone in his family or among his associates who had died of AIDS or was infected with HIV.

2004:

- At a Kimberley election campaign meeting in March, Mbeki justifies the government's slow implementation of the recently-announced ARV rollout programme, saying it would have been 'thoroughly irresponsible' to rush rollout – just as it was irresponsible to build false hopes around ARVs. 'We give people hope that ARVs kill the HI virus. Well, they do not. Why do we tell them that? Why do we do this?'

These incidents of AIDS denialism are taken up again thematically in Part II where their correlation with Cohen's typology of official denial is explored in greater detail. There have been several attempts by AIDS analysts and commentators to explain Mbeki's stance on HIV and AIDS. Most of these analyses point to Mbeki's long exile during apartheid as the source of a paranoid pathology – this, combined with his evident intelligence has led to intellectual conceit on the part of the former President. When questioned or criticised, Mbeki does not hesitate to continually play the race card, accusing detractors of being either the victims of their own Eurocentrism or internalised colonialism, or just blatantly racist. Any opposition to his own points of view are brushed off as being the result of a conspiracy to either unseat him or to counter his own conception of policy problems and public agenda issues in South Africa. This counter-offensive rhetoric at times fits snugly with Cohen's typology of official denial and is subsequently reviewed in our discussion of counter-offensive official denial in Chapter 8. In his actions, however, Mbeki has manifested some paradoxical behaviour to back up his controversial views. Crewe (2000: 10–11) highlights some of these contradictions, noting that:

- In seeking an African solution and to ensure that Western drugs are not relied upon, he will confer with mainly non-Africans for his answer. Indeed many of the [Presidential AIDS P]anel are already collaborators with local programmes and scientists and could give their input via local expertise.
- His government is committed to the development of an HIV vaccine, a full acknowledgement that HIV is the causal connection with AIDS.
- He is aware of the thousands of people who are infected and dying, but refuses to sanction treatment that could reduce this toll.

It is no coincidence, some commentators note, that Mbeki's disastrous foray into the AIDS discourse commenced with the South African government taking on the global pharmaceutical industry in the late 1990s: this battle raged on throughout Mbeki's flirtation with AIDS dissidence and his and his spokespeople's repeated reference to the insidious role that these companies play in South Africa have become a key theme of Mbeki's anti-intellectual rhetoric. According to Sparks (2003: 292):

> it was the dissidents' charges against the pharmaceutical companies that first attracted Mbeki's attention. When [South African dissidents] drew his attention to their websites, Mbeki was himself in the throes of a bitter conflict with these companies...

Some analysts have gone so far as to imply that someone senior in the government might be HIV-positive and so deep in pathological denial that the rest of South Africa has become the victim of irrational thought – Crewe (2001: 125) notes that '[i]t is possible that there is a senior member of government or the ANC who is living with AIDS at a point where the information could be made public'. Denial is also cited by Professor Malegapuru Makgoba (former chairperson of the MRC) who suggests that the government is faced with such a mammoth challenge in the shape of HIV and AIDS that they have been and continue to be grasping at quick fix solutions and explanations (Sparks 2003: 285). When they come across explanations that threaten to expose their own unwillingness to face up the reality of AIDS in South Africa, the very tenets of those arguments are attacked. This might serve to explain Mbeki and some of his Ministers' bizarre questioning of science and scientific methodologies: HIV does not cause AIDS; the MRC and UNAIDS get the statistics wrong; ARVs are toxic and black Africans are being manipulated into using them; racist conspiracies are driving domestic and international opposition against Mbeki's positions; the pharmaceutical companies are bribing South Africa's AIDS civil society, who in turn have infiltrated the ANC's alliance partners. More recently, Makgoba posits a more provocative question (Gill 2006: 72–3). Given the fact that AIDS in South Africa only took off after 1990:

> Did the ANC in addition to bringing liberation also bring AIDS? Nobody wants to address this, and this may be at the heart of the policy difficulty. Members of the liberation army lived in these countries where there was high prevalence. It may explain why there is this denial – that the very movement that brought us freedom might also have brought us something that we don't want to talk about…If I had been in the liberal struggle fighting for freedom and I came back home and suddenly I bring this in addition to liberation, I would react in this way.

Maybe the reality of AIDS was such an insult to Mbeki's dream of an African Renaissance that he would do anything and believe anything in an effort to exculpate African culture or modes of behaviour – going so far as to question the science of AIDS itself (Trengove-Jones 2001: 36). As a private individual, Mbeki was free to believe and advocate what he wishes, but as the head of government of the country with the highest number of HIV-positive citizens in the world, Mbeki was faced with extraordinary responsibilities. His was the responsibility to act swiftly and effectively to counter the spread of HIV, and to ameliorate the impact of AIDS. Public policy and the rollout of effective AIDS programmes fall within the ambit of government responsibility. However, when discussing motives for the Mbeki governments' reactions to the burgeoning epidemic, it is important to consider the epidemic in the context of a long-wave event. As we explore in more detail in Chapter 9, this adds important depth both to considerations of accountability as well as possible motives for official AIDS denial.

That said, there are few who believe that Mbeki and his government were good AIDS managers. In fact, most members of the South African AIDS community point out that Mbeki is guilty of gross negligence (Makgoba 2001) – and this belief is held so strongly that the TAC has even charged his Minister of Health with genocide. According to Schneider (2001: 161) 'the power of political leaders in AIDS lies in three areas: by exerting influence through formal state/government systems, by shaping discourse, and by providing moral authority' – Mbeki clearly failed in all three areas. To make matters worse, Mbeki seemed to not only have gone against the mainstream views of science; he actively sought to redefine the policy problem of AIDS in South Africa itself and acted to exclude anyone outside of government from seizing any opportunity to address the AIDS issue at all (Van der Vliet 2004: 80–81). In doing so, he harmed the efforts of the South African AIDS civil society to keep AIDS on the public agenda. In Mbali's (2003: 322) analysis:

> the denialists have overly prolonged a national debate which has undoubtedly diverted government resources and the attention of government officials from the main policy tasks at hand: using the latest mainstream medical and scientific research to prevent new infections and provide the best standards of care for HIV-infected persons and AIDS orphans.

The President and his Minister of Health acted to delay the implementation of life-saving measures in this country at every possible turn: AIDS civil society in South Africa were continually entangled in legal challenges with the government in an effort to get ARVs and MTCT prevention programmes implemented at public facilities. Until 2006 South Africa had an excellent AIDS policy in the form of the Strategic Plan of 2000. Unfortunately the country's crisis of implementation continued unabatedly. Reflecting on some sectors within government acting autonomously of the executive in efforts to implement AIDS policy, Walker, Reid and Cornell (2004: 125) note that:

> [t]he catapulting of AIDS into the arena of high politics has undoubtedly undermined the ability of the state to mobilise and lead a united response to AIDS in South Africa. However, conflict has tended to occur largely in the political domain and at a national level, involving mainly the Presidency and the health ministry, with the day-to-day bureaucratic realm and provincial governments functioning relatively autonomously and sometimes in contradiction to central political stances.

Mbeki's politicisation of AIDS obfuscated many of the critical messages that his own government's AIDS policy document exemplified – in doing so, Lawrence Schlemmer (quoted in Van der Vliet 2004: 81) suggests that the government and Mbeki were 'shifting blame on history. Campaigns today address risk *behaviour*; linking HIV and AIDS with poverty reverts to a risk *group* analysis, once again stereotyping those at risk'. Some organs of civil society were quite successful in actually bypassing (through litigation) central government's reticence to implement MTCT prevention and ARV programmes. Coupled with a capacitated provincial level of AIDS governance and with radically increased national and provincial AIDS budgets the policy implementers on the ground were in some instances in a position to ignore the noise and obfuscation coming from Mbeki's office. This was of course far from ideal, but the AIDS policy environment seemed to have ceased to be as directly influenced by the Office of the Presidency as it had been earlier.

MTCTP, HAART and the monetarisation of AIDS

The preceding section demonstrates how Mbeki's anti-intellectual or dissident stance damaged the public policy process on HIV and AIDS in South Africa by repeatedly obfuscating the conceptualisation of the policy problem itself. This has had the effect of further confusing the policy agenda, with the government acting on a proclivity to prescribe who has the right to make statements on the epidemic. This has led to the emasculation of the government's own Strategic Plan, rendering it an anachronism in the face of the reality of AIDS. Manning (2001: 106) notes that:

> the debate over the causes of AIDS delayed implementation of a MTCT program, because of the inherent contradiction between administering drugs to prevent HIV transmission while questioning whether HIV causes AIDS; others believe the delay had more to do with limited health sector capacity than with the dissident debate. In any case, the diversion of energy and attention to debates over the cause of AIDS hurt the formulation and implementation of AIDS policy.

The President and his senior health officials muddled AIDS governance by using charges of racism or unfounded conspiracies in an attempt to delegitimise civil society's attempts to create an enabling environment for the implementation of (essentially good) policies. The Mbeki administration's actions (and selective inaction) had three significant consequences: the specific policy problem of treatment became monetarised; in an effort to either bypass the state or to force its hand, some sections of civil society responded by using the strategy of litigation and the artificial separation between prevention (government) and treatment (civil society) response strategies became increasingly politicised and entrenched.

When the Mandela government drafted the *Medicines Bill* of 1997, which led to the PhrMA court case against it, it did so for ostensibly monetary reasons: as noted the state's position was that large pharmaceutical companies were abusing intellectual property provisions in an effort to make obscene profits from the sale of their ARVs and argued that patent rights should not be applied to such an extent that the majority of PWAs in developing countries would be unable to afford appropriate medical treatment. In other words, when the *Medicines Act* of 1998 was first conceived the South African government did not have a problem with the purported toxicity of ARVs. On the contrary, the Mandela government (and then Deputy President Mbeki in particular) was so in favour of their application as a solution to the impact of AIDS that they were pushing for the availability of these drugs. Also, Mbeki was leading the government's effort to register the controversial drug Virodene. Once the drug had been discarded by the medical community, however, Mbeki and those close to him changed their tune: in 1998 the government announced that AZT would no longer be made available to women who had been raped, citing reasons of toxicity and fiscal conservatism. According to Mbali (2003: 317):

> [t]he long-running dispute between civil society and the Government over the efficacy, affordability and safety of anti-retroviral drugs can be traced back to 1998. This was when the National Association of People Living with HIV and AIDS (NAPWA) began to demand that the anti-retroviral AZT be made available to HIV-positive pregnant women to prevent them passing the virus to their children. It was this campaign that led to the formation of the TAC.

However, when faced with evidence to the contrary, namely that ARV drugs or HAART were a safe and essential part of the prevention as well as treatment of AIDS, the Mbeki government increasingly came to use arguments that the drugs were too expensive to provide at public health facilities. To drive their point home the Mbeki government and his Minister of Health joined forces with the TAC in resisting the PhrMA court action and when the international public outcry against the pharmaceutical companies rose to a crescendo in 2001, the PhrMA abandoned their legal action, offered significant reductions in the prices charged for ARVs and even volunteered to provide a few drugs free of charge. In doing so the South African government lost the power afforded by their moral high ground. Their response was not a wholesale embrace of these offers, but rather the government repeated claims that the drugs were unsafe for human consumption and again in the face of solid scientific and econometric proof to the contrary, used the fiscal constraint argument. Despite economists' evidence that it would be more expensive for the South African government *not* to treat PWAs with ARVs the Mbeki government remained steadfast in its refusal to purchase and disseminate these drugs. Government's oscillation between arguments of toxicity and affordability, both in the face of proof to the contrary, makes these likely cases of official denial. Add to this is evidence that government members had financial stakes in Virodene, and possible motives for denial begin to take shape. Thus, in Chapter 7 we discuss arguments of toxicity as a possible instance of interpretive official denial. Monetary arguments are in turn explored as a variant of implicatory official denial.

In March 2000, (Presidential spokesman) Parks Mankahlana off-guardedly justified to *Science* magazine why the South African Department of Health refused to provide a relatively inexpensive [ARV] treatment to pregnant, HIV-positive women: 'That mother is going to die and that HIV-negative child will be an orphan. That child must be brought up. Who is going to bring the child up? It's the state, the state. That's resources, you see' (Bond 2001: 177).

As a consequence to such government opposition, the TAC in particular moved towards increasingly using litigation (or the threat thereof) in an effort to compel the government to provide HAART – particularly in the prevention of MTCT. According to Berger (2001):

> [w]hile the distinguishing feature of public interest litigation in the apartheid area was the attempt to control the exercise of public power and thereby limit and reduce human rights violations, TAC's use of the law in securing access to treatment is to ensure – rather than prevent – state action…[B]y framing political and moral demands in the language of legal rights and constitutional obligations, TAC seeks to use the law without necessarily having to litigate…Litigation is also used to place issues on the agenda, both before the judge and in the court of public opinion.

When the government was defeated, first in the High Court and then in the Constitutional Court, the Minister of Health warned that a dangerous precedent had been set, namely that civil society was using the courts in an effort to circumvent government's powers to determine and implement public policy. Government acted to delay the implementation of the courts' rulings by calling for further studies with regards to the safety of ARVs and then by failing to act in provincial governments' rollout of the Strategic Plan. Again the TAC threatened with court action, leading to great animosity between the TAC-led civil society and the state. Van der Vliet (2004: 75) notes that:

> [p]rovision of nevirapine was patchy, to the extent that in December TAC launched an urgent contempt of court application against the worst offender, Mpumalanga's recalcitrant health MEC, Dr Sibongile Manana, for failing to implement the court order. Tshabalala-Msimang was cited as a second respondent for failing to ensure Manana's compliance.

Importantly, cracks started to appear within the different levels of government, with the ANC's main alliance partners becoming vocal in their disregard for the government's delay tactics: ANC provinces started to rollout HAART and MTCT prevention programmes independently and counter to the wishes of the national Department of Health and the President's office. Furthermore, within the ANC there were calls for the President and senior Department of Health officials to cease their meddling. Late in 2002 the TAC and its partner in the struggle for the implementation of HAART and MTCT prevention programmes, COSATU, used NEDLAC as a forum at which to negotiate (with the government) a strategic plan to roll out MTCT prevention and HAART at a national level. The outcome was successful: a plan was indeed conceptualised, with actuarial scientists noting that the plan could potentially:

- Reduce by nearly 3 million the number of HIV-related deaths between 2002 and 2015.
- Halve the number of children that would otherwise be orphaned by the HIV epidemic by 2015; and
- Produce an average life expectancy in South Africa of approximately 50 years of age as opposed to 40 years in the absence of such interventions (Mbali 2003: 325).

However, soon after the plan was finalised the government refused to sign it, reneging on their undertaking. The TAC and COSATU were so incensed with what they perceived as another effort on the part of the government to delay the implementation of a treatment strategy that they started a national campaign of mass action and continued with legal challenges to the government's reticence to implement policy. In November 2003 the government acquiesced and announced the publication of a strategy to roll out MTCT prevention and HAART programmes, entitled the 'Operational Plan for HIV and AIDS Care and Treatment for South Africa'. Looking back on this, the former head of the government's AIDS Directorate, Dr Nono Simelela, noted that '[w]e got there, but we got there painfully. We bled every step of the way' (Gill 2006: 67). Despite the November 2003 plan, implementation was yet again slow to follow, leading some observers to express a suspicion that the Mbeki government had only announced the rollout strategy in an effort to stave off a popular backlash at the national election in April 2004. As Van der Vliet (2004: 23) notes:

> [t]he November Cabinet decision, even though it has seen precious few people actually receiving ARVs, did serve to draw the sting from HIV and AIDS as an election issue. Voters challenging the government stance could be reassured that treatment was on the way. In the two provinces where the ANC's grip was least secure, the Western Cape and KwaZulu-Natal, health authority initiatives have pre-empted the Minister's glacial rollout delivery.

At the 2003 opening of Parliament over 10,000 demonstrators marched on Parliament in support of the TAC's civil disobedience campaign; in the end, AIDS civil society in South Africa succeeded in garnering sufficient political and popular support for the government to announce a treatment strategy. However, Mbeki has never rescinded his statements casting aspersions on the solid scientific evidence that HIV causes AIDS. The TAC only succeeded in ensuring the drafting of the November 2003 treatment strategy by using mass action and litigation and it was uncertain whether the government would be energetic in implementing the treatment strategy. If the Minister of Health's racist attack in April 2003 on TAC members was anything to go by, the government remained as steadfast as ever in its opposition to any views counter to its own:

> [s]he accused 'a white man' of masterminding the civil disobedience campaign, using Africans, who wait for 'the white man' to deploy them. The attack was obviously directed at TAC's Mark Heywood, who was in the audience. Her repeated reference to 'a white man' eventually led to an angry interchange in which Heywood called the Minister a liar (Van der Vliet 2004: 79).

Unfortunately the civil disobedience campaign did not succeed in countering the erroneous assumption underpinning the government's policy implementation delay tactics, namely that HAART and MTCT prevention strategies are as much part of

AIDS prevention policy as they are of AIDS treatment. The counter-argument is easy to demonstrate and economists and demographers have provided ample evidence of its accuracy: the bottom line is that MTCT prevention and HAART are cost-effective on two main grounds. In the first place they prevent the seroconversion of many newborns, which means that the state would later on have less people to treat for AIDS. In the second place HAART lowers levels of morbidity amongst PWAs, which means that there is less of a burden or demand on the fiscus to respond. PWAs thus remain economically productive for longer, which means that MTCT prevention and HAART strategies to a large extent can pay for themselves.

Mbeki, Part 2: 2004–08

After the April 2004 elections Thabo Mbeki reappointed Manto Tshabalala-Msimang as the Minister of Health. This explicit approval of the Minister's record by the office of the presidency was immediately slammed by the official opposition in Parliament as a 'slap in the face' of PWAs (*Washington Post*, 29 April 2004). The TAC also expressed disappointment with the President's decision, citing the Minister's record of tardy implementation of HIV and AIDS policies. If newspaper reports are to be believed, opposition to Mbeki's decision to reappoint Tshabalala-Msimang also came from within the national Department of Health itself, with the head of the government's AIDS Directorate, Dr Nono Simelela, resigning within weeks of Mbeki's announcement. One year later, reflecting on the Mbeki AIDS initiative, Simelela noted that '[o]ne can't underestimate how much it diverted our attention and slowed us down. They had wasted money. We still hadn't got an answer and people were still dying' (Gill 2006: 63). Within the first month of the Minister's reappointment her historical difficulties in relating to South Africa's AIDS civil society and the broader medical community continued: her department had to face two legal challenges from medical bodies representing South African health care workers, who were unhappy with the directives coming from the health department regarding job specifications with regards to the distribution of drugs.

Any hope of a rapprochement between the Minister and AIDS civil society were dashed during the 15th International AIDS Conference, which was held in Bangkok in July 2004. Tshabalala-Msimang reacted badly to suggestions from then UN Secretary General Kofi Annan's Special Envoy on HIV and AIDS in Africa, Dr Stephen Lewis, that the South African government was 'dragging its feet' on the rollout of ARVs. The Minister accused Lewis – despite his numerous visits to South Africa – of being ignorant about the South African epidemic. This context of animosity at the Bangkok conference was made worse by the Minister's continued questioning of the efficacy and safety of the use of the ARV drug Nevirapine for the purpose of preventing MTCT. Despite evidence to the contrary the Minister repeated her oft-stated claims that the drug was toxic and that its application for MTCT prevention was irresponsible. The public spat between the Minister and the TAC over this issue dominated the rest of the Bangkok conference. The situation was exacerbated when the Minister – citing official obligations in South Africa – decided to leave Bangkok after attending the conference for only one day. This led to members of South Africa's AIDS civil society again questioning Tshabalala-Msimang's commitment to the fight against the epidemic.

After the Bangkok conference the battle between the health department and the TAC escalated. Since the announcement of the government's Treatment Plan in November 2003 the TAC had been struggling to get access to the government's timetable for the actual implementation of this latest policy venture. Citing the government's failure to implement its stated intentions to have 53,000 HIV-positive South Africans on ARV treatment by March 2004 (the government had by October 2004 only succeeded in rolling out such treatment to 15,000 PWAs) the TAC in November 2004 once again turned to the courts to force the government to make public its proposed treatment schedule. This time the TAC hoped to invoke the *Open Democracy Act*, which guarantees South Africans the right to view the contents of all public (government) documents.

Mbeki also came under fire for his continued silence on the AIDS epidemic. In October 2004 the official opposition's spokesperson on health during official question time in Parliament asked Mbeki whether the government was not concerned that the high incidence of rape in South Africa is fuelling the AIDS epidemic. Mbeki refused to answer the question, instead attacking the spokesperson and the official opposition in a thinly veiled attempt to (once again) emphasise the fact that racism was a bigger problem for South Africans. After that Mbeki again was criticised by the media and other policy actors, who accused the President of once again attempting to monopolise the right to determine the policy agenda. In addition, Archbishop Desmond Tutu was in late November 2004 involved in a public spat with Mbeki after the Archbishop questioned what he saw as the culture of sycophancy within the ruling party and Mbeki's reticence to answer questions regarding AIDS amongst other issues. This led to acrimonious exchanges between Tutu and ANC spokespeople, as well as directly with the President. Mbeki was also criticised for not owing up to South Africa's bad track record on sexual violence. In October 2004 Mbeki launched a scathing attack on journalist Charlene Smith and UNAIDS's Deputy Director, Kathleen Cravero, for emphasising the need in the country to address the issue of rape. Such emphases were in Mbeki's analysis really just racist attempts to discredit the new South Africa.

In December 2004 elements within the ANC also repeated their earlier attacks on the TAC, namely that the organisation was in bed with large pharmaceutical companies and using poor South Africans as guinea pigs in a ploy to distribute toxic drugs to the indigent (*ANC Today* 17 December 2004). The TAC hit back by pointing out that the government was trying to detract attention from the fact that by the end of 2004 fewer than 20,000 people in the public sector were on ARV therapy while more than 45,000 people in the private sector had access to ARVs:

> Those of us who can afford to have the chance to live, while poor and mainly black people die because of bureaucratic neglect. A section of the ANC

> leadership frequently misuses the allegation of racisim to cover up mistakes or lies (*News24.com*, 18 January 2005).

To drive their point home, the government around the same time pointed out that the South African National Blood Service (SANBS) was still applying outdated racist criteria in deciding which blood donations to accept: the SANBS until early 2005 was excluding the serum of black people, since such blood had been found to contain high levels of HIV. The vitriol that resulted from this revelation of racial profiling in the health services eventually led to the institution of a more expensive but racially blind system to make the South African blood supply safer. However, this positive outcome was clouded by the reracialising of the issue of the national blood supply, providing the government with an opportunity to deflect attention from their slack rollout of ARV treatment. (Ironically – despite the fact that the South African epidemic is chiefly heterosexually established – in January 2006 the SANBS announced that blood from homosexual men would (again) be excluded).

In January 2005 this context of contestation became even more political when the head of the Catholic Bishops Conference in Southern Africa, Cardinal Wilfred Napier, criticised the government for promoting condoms in the fight against HIV and AIDS 'when it's clearly not working' (*News24.com*, 24 January 2005). Confusing theology with sociology, the Catholic Church used the most recent AIDS fracas in an attempt to drive their own anachronistic and moralistic agenda – at the expense of tried and tested methods for preventing the spread of HIV. By the end of January 2005 the health department admitted that their ARV rollout programme was lagging. The national Department of Health's new Director for HIV and AIDS, Dr Nomonde Xundu, reported that only 33,000 people with full-blown AIDS were receiving free drugs by the end of that month. Xundu noted that the department's biggest challenge was to get the human resources capacity up to the level where it needs to be – the health department set a goal of hiring 220 doctors by March 2005, but only 111 had been found. Also, out of the 271 pharmacists needed to help roll out the ARV treatment programme only 90 were hired and only 64 of the 136 dieticians required were hired. Members of AIDS civil society reacted to this admission by saying that missed targets were rooted in a lack of political will from a government whose leader has in the past openly shown his scepticism over the need to make the fight against the AIDS epidemic a priority. Responding to the 2005–06 national budget allocation to health, these activists also criticised the government for not keeping up with inflation or with health practitioners' salaries and for focusing so exclusively on the expansion of health infrastructure that inadequate planning went into expanding the actual delivery of services where they were needed.

One of the most significant developments in the world of HIV and AIDS in South Africa occurred in February 2005, when the South African Medical Research Council announced national mortality figures for the country. The data showed that deaths amongst adults had risen by around 60 per cent between 1997 and 2003 and the researchers concluded that the under-reporting of deaths related to AIDS was the greatest cause for this increase. An editorial in the eminent international journal *The Lancet* (12 February 2005) used this information to lambast the Mbeki government for its continued denialism and foot-dragging on the rollout of ARV drugs:

> Social stigma associated with HIV and AIDS, tacitly perpetuated by the government's reluctance to bring the crisis out in the open and face it head on, prevents many from speaking out about causes of illness and deaths of loved ones and leads doctors to record uncontroversial diagnoses on death certificates…The South African government needs to stop being defensive and show backbone and courage to acknowledge and seriously tackle the HIV and AIDS crisis of its people. The progress in provision of [ARV] treatment to all people with advanced HIV has been painfully slow since the Government's first report of a planned programme in August 2003.

Despite this potentially explosive information the government seemed to be continuing its intransigent position on ARVs and continued to prevaricate on the rollout of ARV treatments. The Minister of Health remained obstinate in her refusal to endorse the use of ARVs. Instead, her (some would say irresponsible and genocidal) advocacy of olive oil, lemon, the African potato and garlic as serious alternatives to ARVs were finding dangerous footholds in her department's support for controversial figures such as Matthias Rath, a German doctor who strongly opposes ARVs and promotes vitamins as a treatment for AIDS and other diseases. The Minister met with Rath in April 2005 and after that his South African endeavours received a generous measure of protection from the government. Such behaviour from the Minister was taken as an indication that senior members of the South African government remained firmly ensconced in a denialist mindset – to illustrate this, journalist Peter Gill reported on a conversation he had with the Minister in 2005 (Gill 2006: 70):

> I thought I should establish whether the government had moved on from the 'denialism' that characterised the first Mbeki term. Untreated HIV leads to AIDS, doesn't it? [he asked the Minister]. 'Not necessarily', the Minister replied. 'There are people who live for 20 or 25 years, and they do not have AIDS-defining illness'. Only insignificant numbers, surely? 'But some of them get ill for a time, they manage their illness, and they're fine again. You can't say it leads necessarily to AIDS'.

Clearly the 'high political' AIDS terrain in South Africa remained contested and in disarray deep into the second Mbeki administration. Every day nearly 1,000 South Africans were dying and nearly 1,500 South Africans were becoming infected with the HI virus – unnecessarily. This contested high political arena was thus having very real effects in the low politics of the every day management of HIV and AIDS in South Africa. Here follow a few illustrations:

- In October 2005 the Department of Finance announced that the Health Department was unable to spend R67.2 million that had been budgeted for AIDS projects in the preceding financial year; the Minister of Health blamed provincial governments and NGOs for not effectively monitoring the spending of the conditional grant from central government.
- In November 2005 Stephen Lewis, then UN Secretary General Kofi Annan's special AIDS envoy for Africa, said that the South African Minister of Health was preventing him from doing his job in this country; he also accused South Africa of acting more slowly than poorer countries such as Lesotho and Malawi in rolling out ARV programmes. Later in that month the UN announced that 85 per cent of South Africans in need of ARVs had still not received them by mid-2005; the Department of Health responded by blaming government inaction before 1994 as the main reason why AIDS has not been curbed.
- At the opening of Parliament in February 2006 Thabo Mbeki mentioned AIDS only once. Later in the month, the TAC singled out Mbeki and the Minister of Health in a report to the NEPAD African Peer Review Mechanism for failing to respond to the AIDS epidemic.
- In May 2006 the government announced that 134,473 HIV-positive South Africans were on ARVs provided for at public facilities by the end of March. (More than 500,000 South Africans remained in need of ARVs).
- In the same month the government first excluded the TAC from a national delegation to attend a United Nations AIDS summit in New York in early June.
- At the UN summit the South African government came under criticism from the African Civil Society Coalition on AIDS for undermining a continent-wide African position committing African nations to firm numerical targets to counter the AIDS epidemic – the targets had been agreed one month before at a meeting of the AU in West Africa.
- Later in June 2006 the South African government announced that they wanted large AIDS donors to channel all funding through the state rather than funding AIDS civil society directly. This led to an outcry of opposition from members of AIDS NGOs and CBOs.
- In July 2006 the Department of Health released the latest AIDS epidemic data for South Africa. The data again indicated a marginal increase in national AIDS prevalence. Whereas the Department of Health emphasised the fact that the epidemic seemed to be stabilising, other experts (including Dr Olive Shisana, former Director General of the Health Department and now the head of the Human Sciences Research Council) noted that this was probably simply due to higher mortality (death) rates in the country and that incidence levels remained shockingly high, indicating that the epidemic was still not retreating in South Africa.

Reviewing these events after the second Mbeki administration came to power in April 2004 and until July 2006 it is clear that the negative patterns of public rhetoric and actions on HIV and AIDS established during 1999–2004 were continuing. Negative aspects centred around the fact that Mbeki and his Minister of Health were continuing their mixed messages and foot-dragging on ARV rollout. Government continued to question medical science, cast doubt on any data demonstrating the affordability and imperative of life-saving drugs, or the negative impact that AIDS is having on national mortality and morbidity levels. This overview also illustrates quite clearly that signs of government denial at the time went far beyond the ambit of scientific AIDS denialism. When viewed against Cohen's typology, the political overtones in this intensifying rhetoric of blame suggest that denial was deeply rooted in government's response to the epidemic. This is explored in more detail in the ensuing discussion.

August 2006 to June 2007: Rehabilitating Mbeki's AIDS governance?

After July 2006 a number of significant developments in the South African HIV and AIDS environment occurred which many hoped would introduce a new era of co-operation and constructive engagement amongst the important AIDS stakeholders in South Africa. These changes resulted from the chaos that exemplified South Africa's official participation at the 16th Global AIDS Conference that was held in Toronto in August 2006. At the conference the South African Department of Health's stall consisted of a display of garlic, lemons and beetroot, with two bottles of ARVs hastily added after complaints. The TAC delegation at the conference physically attacked and disassembled the stall and again criticised the Minister of Health, who at later news conferences reiterated her controversial position that good nutrition can be an alternative to ARVs.

During the closing ceremony of the conference the UN secretary general's Special Envoy on AIDS in Africa, Dr Stephen Lewis, lambasted the South African government for its mismanagement of the AIDS epidemic. A few weeks after the conference 82 of the most prominent AIDS scholars in the world sent a letter to President Mbeki asking him to relieve Health Minister Tshabalala-Msimang of her duties (letter to Mbeki 4 September 2006). During the same month the government was censured in the Durban High Court for dragging its feet in providing ARVs to prisoners in a KwaZulu-Natal prison; the case had been brought against the government by representatives of the AIDS Law Project, who represented the prisoners. Also, it was reported in the media that the Minister of Health had given orders to her Deputy, Dr Nozizwe Madlala-Routledge, that the latter was not to make any public statements regarding HIV and AIDS – it was well known that the Minister and the Deputy Minister of Health did not see eye to eye on the government's handling of the epidemic.

In the last few months of 2006 the Minister of Health was taken ill and went on prolonged sick leave. In her absence the government appointed Deputy President Phumzile Mlambo-Ncquka, in her capacity as the chairperson of SANAC, as well as the Deputy Minister of Health as the custodians of governmental AIDS management. The two politicians, who are known to hold positions on HIV and AIDS that are contrary to the Minister of Health's, immediately started to consult with members of South Africa's AIDS civil society. In the absence of Minister Tshabalala-Msimang the national AIDS response moved to embrace a more traditional biomedical view of the epidemic, committed themselves to a speedy rollout of ARVs and moved to redesigning the national Strategic AIDS Plan in conjunction with government's former foes, the TAC as well as other civil society groups.

Emboldened by international support as well as government statements that were more in line with their own, members of civil society expressed their willingness to engage with the offices of the 'two deputies' and by the end of the year the national Department of Health was able to advance the drafting of the new Strategic Plan in an environment almost wholly devoid of the contestation that had been so emblemic of public AIDS management in South Africa in recent years. By February 2007 the Minister of Health (after a brief return to office) went on further sick leave and the Minister of Transport (a member of the government who is known for his mainline, anti-denialist AIDS position) was appointed as acting Health Minister. In March 2007 the Department of Health launched their draft *HIV and AIDS and STI Strategic Plan: 2007–2011*. The Plan, which found great support amongst all the main AIDS actors in the country, was officially submitted to SANAC at the end of March 2007. During the launch the acting Minister made a point of emphasising the 'spirit of renewed partnership among all the role-players in the response to HIV and AIDS' (Radebe 14 March 2007).

The HIV and AIDS and STI Strategic Plan: 2007–11

When the Department of Health embarked on its course to redesign the National Strategic Plan (NSP) of 2000–05 it first identified the main weaknesses of the existing AIDS strategy. The NSP of 2000 gave rise to the establishment and expansion of key programmes such as health education, voluntary HIV counselling and testing (VCT), prevention of mother-to-child transmission (MTCT) and anti-retroviral therapy (ART). There had been some growth in input to and uptake of these programmes over the period of the NSP 2000–05. However, the implementation of these programmes tended to be vertical, with capacity deficits evident in their implementation. This was taken as reflective of the health system or lead agency's weaknesses rather than as a weakness in the strategic framework. The lack of a clear monitoring and evaluation (M&E) framework and clear targets and responsibilities had been a major weakness of the NSP 2000–05, as was the overall co-ordination of activities at SANAC level and within civil society.

In May 2006 the SANAC under the leadership of its chairperson Deputy President Mlambo-Ngcuka mandated the health department to lead a process of developing a new five-year NSP for the years 2007–11. The *HIV and AIDS and STI Strategic Plan for South Africa: 2007–11* (see Table 6.2) flows from the *National Strategic Plan of 2000–05* as well as the *Operational Plan for Comprehensive HIV and AIDS Care, Management and Treatment* (November 2003). It represents the country's multisectoral response to the challenge with HIV infection and the wide-ranging impacts of AIDS. The process of redesigning the NSP started with a rapid assessment of the implementation of the NSP 2000–05. In September 2006 a report of the assessment highlighted the following findings:

- All stakeholders embraced the NSP 2000–05 as a guiding framework.
- It served to broaden the involvement of agencies beyond the health department and gave rise to the establishment and expansion of key programmes such as health education, voluntary counselling and testing (VCT), mother-to-child transmission prevention (MTCTP) and anti-retroviral therapy (ART).
- However, stigma and discrimination remained unacceptably high and this as a deterrent to the utilisation of some of the services.
- Also, implementation of programmes tended to be vertical, with some serious capacity deficits especially in rural communities; and

Table 6.2 Outline of the HIV and AIDS and STI Strategic Plan for South Africa: 2007–11

The key guiding principles:
Supportive leadership
Effective communication
Effective partnerships
Promoting social change and cohesion
Sustainable programmes and funding
The primary goals are to:
Reduce the number of new HIV infections by 50 per cent
Reduce the impact of HIV and AIDS on individuals, families, communities and society by expanding access to appropriate treatment, care and support to 80 per cent of all people diagnosed with HIV
Four main areas constitute the Strategic Plan:
1. Prevention
Goal 1: Reduce vulnerability to HIV infection and the impact of AIDS
Goal 2: Reduce sexual transmission of HIV
Goal 3: Reduce mother-to-child transmission of HIV
Goal 4: Minimise the risk of HIV transmission through blood and blood products

Table 6.2 Continued

Goal 3: Reduce mother-to-child transmission of HIV
Goal 4: Minimise the risk of HIV transmission through blood and blood products
2. Treatment, care and support
Goal 5: Increase coverage of voluntary counseling and testing and promote regular HIV testing
Goal 6: Enable people living with HIV to lead healthy and productive lives
Goal 7: Address the special needs of women and children
Goal 8: Mitigate impacts of HIV and AIDS and create an enabling social environment for care, treatment and support
3. Research, monitoring and surveillance
Goal 9: Implement the monitoring and evaluation framework of the NSP
Goal 10: Support the development of prevention technologies
Goal 11: Support AIDS vaccine development
Goal 12: Conduct operational research
Goal 13: Conduct policy research
Goal 14: Conduct regular surveillance
4. Human rights, access to justice and law reform
Goal 15: Ensure knowledge of and adherence to the existing legal and policy frameworks
Goal 16: Mobilise society and build leadership of people living with HIV to protect and promote human rights
Goal 17: Identify and remove legal, policy, and cultural barriers to effective HIV prevention, treatment and support
Goal 18: Mobilise society to respect and protect human rights of women and girls, including those with disabilities, to eradicate gender-based violence and advance equality in sexual relationships

- The two major weaknesses of the NSP 2000–05 were poor co-ordination at the level of SANAC as well as lack of clear targets and a monitoring framework.

Key recommendations included a need:

- For a revision of the behaviour change approaches.
- To strengthen government implementation.
- Tonsolidate and build existing partnerships.
- To trengthen co-ordination, monitoring and evaluation at the level of SANAC.
- To increase the contribution of the business sector, especially with regard to SMMEs; and

- To make all interventions accessible to people with disabilities.

In addition, key features of the *New Strategic Plan 2007–11* included:

- A mandate for the health department and research institutions to measure progress towards reaching these goals.
- The creation of a special unit in the health department to monitor the plan's implementation.
- A mid-term review scheduled for 2009; and
- Specific, quantified targets, including:
  - Providing treatment to 80 per cent of the adults who need it by 2011.
  - Reducing the proportion of adults starting ART in hospitals to 30 per cent; and
  - Increasing the number of HIV patients on treatment overseen by nurses to 70 per cent.

June 2007 to September 2008: In with the old, out with the new

Unfortunately the positive changes in the South African AIDS governance environment came to an abrupt end with the return from sick leave in June 2007 of Minister of Health Manto Tshabalala-Msimang. The Minister immediately moved to reassert her power in the Ministry of Health, as well as over the management of AIDS in South Africa. The open lines of communication between AIDS civil society and the government that were put in place during the Minister's absence were shut down and the Minister made a point of restating her opposition to the use of ARVs in the treatment of AIDS. She again advocated her long-held belief in garlic, lemon rind, the African potato and other vegetables as alternatives to AIDS drugs, rather than viewing good nutrition as complementary to the medication. The Minister also still supported the activities of Dr Matthias Rath, who marketed vitamins as an alternative to ARVs.

Significantly, the Minister acted to rein in her Deputy, Dr Nozizwe Madlala-Routledge, who was ordered to stop speaking publically about HIV and AIDS, and to limit her public profile. The Deputy Minister then made the 'errors' of having a public AIDS test, speaking openly with the TAC, promoting access to ARV treatment, and of visiting a public hospital in the Eastern Cape province and then speaking to the media about the poor conditions there. This angered the Minister and the President, who insisted that Madlala-Routledge resign due to what was presented to her as her lack of loyalty. The Deputy Minister refused to resign and informed Mbeki that if he wanted to get rid of her, he would have to fire her. On 8 August 2007 Thabo Mbeki did just that, using a dubious technicality (the Deputy Health Minister's purportedly unauthorised attendance of an international AIDS conference) to relieve her of her duties. On 12 August 2007 Madlala-Routledge went public with the real dynamics surrounding her dismissal, prompting an intellectualised tirade of disapproval from Mbeki in his subsequent weekly online newsletter. This attempt at (falsely) constructing the Deputy Minister as someone who was corrupt and attempting to undermine the authority of higher-ranking officials resonates with Cohen's description of counter-offensive denial and will be discussed as such later in Chapter 8.

AIDS denialism was also back in the saddle: vitamin salesman Matthias Rath was still supported by the Minister of Health, despite a court judgment on 13 June 2008 which found that the state had failed to enforce its own legislation to control medical trials without the approval of the Medical Controls Council. The Minister also, in January 2008, cast the only dissenting vote at the National Health Council on a revised protocol on MTCTP – despite a Constitutional Court order in 2002 permitting such a protocol. The health department also continued to sanction medical health officers who used donor funds to implement the MTCTP protocol. The TAC and the ALP were persistent in using the law and human rights in defending these doctors, and in the end the courts consistently condemned government's actions. However, as Heywood (2009: 18–19) notes, 'what is worrying is the pattern of largely unchecked government misconduct that emerges from these cases, casting serious doubt on the executive's respect for the rule of law'. By mid-2007 donors and members of AIDS civil society were explicit that they despaired at any possibility of sensible, constructive AIDS governance in South Africa as long as Mbeki and Tshabalala-Msimang continued to be in government (Fourie, Perche and Schoeman 2010).

In the end, the African National Congress agreed with this sentiment. In December 2007 Thabo Mbeki was replaced as party President by Jacob Zuma and on 20 September 2008 the ANC fired Mbeki as head of state for abusing the criminal justice system in an attempt to keep Zuma from challenging Mbeki's leadership. Ironically, this was eight years to the day after Mbeki infamously stated in Parliament that HIV does not cause AIDS. On 25 September 2008 Barbara Hogan replaced Tshabalala-Msimang as Minister of Health, and soon after announced that 'the era of AIDS denialism is over completely in South Africa' (quoted in Dugger 2008).

Sadly, Mbeki's failings on AIDS will probably dominate his legacy. The Harvard study mentioned earlier (Chigwedere et al. 2008) stated in December 2008 that Mbeki's inaction to provide ARVs to South Africans living with the HI virus in the years between 2000 and 2005 cost more than 330,000 lives, with 35,000 babies born HIV-positive because of delays in the provision of MTCTP drugs. According to Chigwedere et al. (2008: 410) '[t]he total lost benefits of ARVs are at least 3.8 million person-years for the period 2000–2005'. Importantly, the study does not include the numbers of people between 2005 and 2008 – and the numbers that are available are based on conservative assumptions; the real number is probably much worse. Max Essex, the virologist who has led Harvard's AIDS research programme since the early days of the global pandemic, called South Africa's response to AIDS under Thabo Mbeki 'a case of bad, or even evil, public health' (quoted in Dugger 2008).

PART II
Making Sense of Official AIDS Denial

Now that we have told the story of successive South African governments' responses to AIDS, from the early 1980s to the end of the Mbeki era, we turn to investigating the suspected instances of official denial that were highlighted in the preceding discussion. In other words, as noted earlier, in Part II (Chapters 7–10) we change our analytical focus from a 'what' to a 'how and why' investigation into the theory of South African AIDS denial that was formulated in Chapter 3. Part II therefore breaks the historical narrative of Part I into themes, for the sake of analytical clarity.

In the next two chapters we apply Stanley Cohen's typology of official denial to the possible cases of government denial that were pointed out in the preceding historical narrative of the South African government's handling of the epidemic. As outlined in Chapter 3, Cohen's typology deals with three broad categories of official denial: classic official denial (literal, interpretive and implicatory), counter-offensive denial and partial acknowledgement. Applying Cohen's typology provides an opportunity to validate, (at least in theory) whether these suspected cases of denial can in fact be considered official denial. By introducing Cohen's typology a picture thus begins to develop that should shed more light on the frequency and intensity of this suspected government denial.

With the added insight offered by epidemiology and the study of long-wave events, in Chapter 9 we are then able to point out probable underlying political motives and trends that may have informed South African official denial during the epidemic. This discussion also touches on the dynamics of blame, accountability, victimhood and the construction of bogeymen in the history of AIDS in South Africa.

To conclude our discussion, in Chapter 10 we turn our attention once more to a historical overview. By mapping the possible cases of official denial we have indentified using Cohen's typology, against a timeline of the epidemic, we are able to sketch a theme of denial that appears to have persisted (albeit subtly at times) throughout the course of the epidemic. Finally, we summarise our key findings and propose areas for future research.

Chapter 7
Classic Official Denial

Before embarking on a more detailed look at government denial, it is important to note that the mechanisms of denial are varied and can be highly flexible. As Cohen (2001: 103) points out, officials often use a number of forms of denial in order to diffuse a situation. One incident can therefore often be classified under a variety of categories within the typology. When engaging in a public relations battle relating to a controversy, officials' rhetoric may therefore exhibit a number of elements of official denial. These strategies could also be used in sequence with officials reverting, for instance, to interpretive denial if initial approaches using literal denial failed or were exposed (Cohen 2001: 103).

As official denial is most frequently found in government rhetoric, in the following two chapters particular cases of suspected denial are identified by headings that summarise the argument used by the officials. To emphasise the strong communicative or rhetorical element in these strategies, the headings are crafted in quote form to represent the message government officials appear to have conveyed through their actions and statements. This is meant to continually create awareness of the manner in which official denial tends to be embedded in the public relations material of a government.

This chapter is the first of two in which Stanley Cohen's typology of official denial is applied to the history of South African AIDS governance in order to investigate the theory of official denial we have outlined in Chapter 3. Taken together, the next two chapters cover the three broad categories of official denial contained in Cohen's typology: classic official denial, counter-offensive denial and partial acknowledgement. Whilst classic official denial tends to be more blatant, the latter two forms of denial are subtler. Classic official denial thus presents a more traditional kind of government denial that deals with the three basic types of denial as outlined Chapter 3: literal denial, interpretive denial and implicatory denial.

Literal official denial

Literal denial is based on the assertion that 'nothing happened' or 'nothing is wrong'. It involves denying, literally, that an event occurred or is occurring at all. Maintaining such a position of complete ignorance is extremely problematic in democratic states with a free press. This tactic is therefore most characteristic of authoritarian and repressive regimes (Cohen 2001: 104). It should therefore come as no surprise that most of the instances that could be construed as literal denial are drawn from the apartheid era.

'AIDS only kills homosexuals, commercial sex workers and intravenous drug users'

The apartheid policy makers' initial response to the emerging epidemic is perhaps the most consistent with literal official denial. When the first two AIDS deaths were reported in South Africa in 1982 the state's initial response was 'to quell any possible panic reactions amongst the white public and to assure them that they were in no danger' (Grundlingh 2001: 125). In so doing the Department of Health made two statements that would put the general public at ease. First, Dr J. Gillard, Director General of the Department of Health, announced that the public was not at risk as the virus was confined mostly to white gay men. A few days later the Department of Health proceeded to point out that the two men who had died of the disease could have been isolated cases (Grundlingh 2001: 125).

By framing AIDS as a homosexual issue and as a largely isolated one at that, the government managed to set up a convenient scapegoat that allowed them to pay very little heed to the emerging epidemic in its early years. Later, commercial sex workers and intravenous drug users were added to the ranks of homosexuals as the primary carriers of AIDS. As the virus was still confined to an 'expendable' cohort and not the 'general public' it continued to be an issue of little concern to the government and therefore remained easy to disregard (Grundlingh 2001: 126). In fact, the Department of Health only mentioned AIDS in its annual report in 1985 – three years after the first two AIDS deaths had been recorded. Even then the mention of AIDS continued to be framed as isolated, mostly white homosexual cases. The 1985 report stressed that all 21 diagnosed cases of AIDS were male of which 16 were gay, three heterosexual and one bisexual. Moreover, the three heterosexual cases were crafted as having some connection with Zaire (today the Democratic Republic of the Congo). The final listed infection was the result of blood transfusion. Of the 21 cases, 20 were white (Furlong and Ball 2005: 129).

These reactions are strongly reminiscent of Cohen's description of literal official denial as a means of telling the public 'nothing is wrong'. Presenting AIDS as a disease that posed no real threat to the majority of 'normal' South Africans not only gave it a greater foothold in society (as its spread was virtually unchecked in those initial years), but also laid the foundations for a culture of taboo and stigmatisation that has come to characterise the AIDS issue.[1] Moreover, the depiction of AIDS as confined to these marginal groups who at the time were predominantly white, created the dangerous misperception amongst black South Africans that they were not at risk.

It is important, however, to acknowledge the very incremental onset of the epidemic. Today, with the necessary hindsight, the apartheid government's disregard of the situation is placed in a much more serious light than it may have appeared at the time. Also, knowledge of the disease in those early years was limited and ignorance was a major contributing factor to government inaction

1 As Altman (2006) points out, many of the taboos around HIV and AIDS have their roots in the history of the epidemic and in particular in officials' dealings with it at the time.

not only in South Africa, but the world over. This makes any certain statement that government was in blatant denial problematic. Nonetheless, there is some correlation between these early government statements and what Cohen describes as literal denial.

'AIDS is a black disease'

As the epidemic progressed, so did awareness of the situation. Towards the mid-to-late 1980s it became apparent that AIDS in South Africa had made that transition from homosexuals to heterosexuals. As we pointed out in Chapter 4, the growing urgency of the situation did not, however, result in any significant changes in government action or rhetoric. Instead, the issue was projected on the broader racialised context of the day and the by now clearly escalating situation continued to be marginalised. Although the apartheid government began to acknowledge the AIDS 'problem', they approached the issue in a manner that strongly suggested that AIDS was a black disease and therefore posed no threat to the white population (the only real demographic group that was of interest to the ruling party). Officials effectively turned what was initially the 'gay plague' into the 'black death' as they went from constructing AIDS as an issue of moral deviance to one of race.

This was particularly evident in the apartheid government's warnings that ANC cadres would bring the virus back upon their return from exile in other African countries. The belief that AIDS affected only the black population was so strongly embedded that, it has been rumoured, National Party (NP) canvassers assured white voters that black majority rule did not pose a threat as AIDS would soon virtually exterminate all black South Africans. In response, an MP from the South African Conservative Party replied, 'it would be like Father Christmas' if AIDS ended black population growth (Van der Vliet 2001: 156). Alarmingly, this macabre hope for the extermination of black South Africans indicates that at least some members of government were well aware of the destructive potential of the epidemic. And yet the government had so successfully embedded their conception of the epidemic as marginalised to expendable groups in society (blacks, gays, prostitutes and drug addicts) that some policy makers seemed quite happy to welcome this plague into the country.

Whilst whites were assured of a black decimation, the black communities, thanks to the initial selling of the epidemic as limited to white homosexuals, largely discounted warnings of a heterosexual plague. In this climate of oppression and political manipulation, conspiracy theories flourished. An article in the ANC publication *Sechaba* mused that AIDS was part of an imperialist plot to undermine anti-apartheid activism (Van der Vliet 2001: 156). Other popular theories considered the possibility that AIDS was a deception employed by the apartheid government to discourage procreation amongst black people. And so the 'black' explanation for the acronym AIDS was coined: *A*frikaner *I*nvention to *D*iscourage *S*ex. Whilst the 'black' understanding of AIDS cannot be considered a deliberate attempt at denial by the government, it does illustrate the (often unintended) consequences that government propaganda can have.

It is possible that government denial of AIDS during this time was simply a function of the overall ethos of denial that the apartheid government fostered and enforced. On this basis it could be argued that homosexuals and black citizens were already treated with a great deal of denial and that this denial of their right to health was more an extension of existing government denial than deliberate and blatant AIDS denial.

'AIDS is not the biggest killer, crime is'

In a modern, democratic system it is increasingly difficult for officials to maintain positions of literal denial. Increased international visibility and transparency have made these blatantly deceptive manoeuvres difficult to sustain (Cohen 2001: 105). Literal denial has therefore seldom featured in the post-apartheid South African government's box of rhetorical tricks – with the exception of government-sponsored AIDS denialism. As it is essentially characterised by an outright defiance of medial and scientific fact, AIDS denialism is a classic example of literal denial. Thabo Mbeki, as the notorious champion of denialism, therefore is a key actor in the following two cases of official literal denial.

During his first term of office, Mbeki found himself frequently at odds with official statistics regarding South Africans' cause of death. In an interview with the BBC (August 2001) Mbeki maintained that crime and violence were the country's main cause of mortality (and not AIDS). On these grounds he then urged a revision of government AIDS policy, using seven-year old WHO statistics to argue that AIDS should be a minor concern to government. In a subsequent letter to the Minister of Health he maintained that people who consider AIDS the 'single biggest cause of death' have 'convinced themselves' of this fact and that government policy and programmes should not be 'informed by misperceptions' about AIDS (see Chapter 6).

A month later, a Medical Research Council (MRC) cause-of-death study was leaked to the media that clearly refuted Mbeki's claims. The report testified to the outdatedness of the WHO statistics and confirmed that AIDS was still, in fact, the biggest cause of adult mortality in South Africa. The Office of the President, however, showed little faith in the MRC report, delaying its official release and expressing doubts about its credibility. Mbeki's public refusal to acknowledge the (scientifically demonstrable) toll taken by AIDS is a classic example of literal denial. Contesting the major cause of death in South Africa in the face of credible evidence is, by its very definition, denial. Essentially literal denial of this kind characterises AIDS denialism. Cause of death statistics are particularly menacing for denialists as they have the potential to disprove many of their arguments. Typically denialists challenge the accuracy of these figures by arguing that the recorded increase of deaths are either due to poverty or improved data collection methods (Nattrass 2007: 94).

'...and besides, do we even know what causes AIDS?'

Mbeki's grappling with the causes of AIDS is another very likely case of literal official denial. At times he questioned 'the "paradigm" of AIDS' (Gevisser 2007: 729), expressing doubt that the collapse of the immune system is caused by the HI virus. In June 2000, whilst opening the 13th International AIDS Conference in Durban, Mbeki suggested that poverty rather than HIV was responsible for AIDS deaths in South Africa. He has also argued that a virus (HIV) cannot cause a syndrome (AIDS).

Interpretive official denial

As a second variant of classic official denial, apart from blatantly denying fact, officials can admit to the raw facts of a wrongdoing but provide their own interpretation that differs from the mainstream, conventional one in an attempt to absolve them from responsibility or blame. Effectively they would be arguing that 'what is happening is really something else' (Cohen 2001: 105). This approach is known as interpretive official denial and it is the second of the three forms of classic official denial identified by Cohen. Employing interpretive official denial in the case of AIDS could, for instance entail acknowledging the HIV and AIDS epidemic ('ok, so we have an AIDS problem...'), but then seek ways to diffuse the situation, make it look less threatening, or blame someone or something else for it ('...but it is confined to deviant members of society'; or '...this is apartheid's fault'). Cohen (2001: 106) calls this 'cognitively reframing harm' with the utility of relocating it to 'a different, less pejorative class of event'. Part of this tactic also involves policy makers dressing up the issue in a manner that would allow them to argue that the situation is not what it appears to be (Cohen 2001: 105). This could include arguments like: 'ARVs are not life-saving treatment, they are toxic', 'it is poverty and not a virus that causes AIDS', or in the case of the apartheid governments, 'AIDS does not really affect white people'.

There are a number of variations of interpretive denial that often charatcerise policy makers' rhetoric. Officials may invoke *euphemism* to make an issue appear less dire than it is. Or they could resort to the discipline and discourse of law to diffuse a situation. This is known as *legalism*. They may also devise a scapegoat and then *deny responsibility*. Or they could admit to an act or a situation, accept responsibility, but argue that it is an *isolated event* (Cohen 2001: 107–9). A number of incidences in South African policy makers' responses resonate strongly with these manoeuvres.

'Only a few homosexuals, commercial sex workers and drug users are affected'

Isolation was a key element of one of the first responses of South African policy makers to the epidemic. As mentioned in Chapter 4, shortly after the first two AIDS deaths were recorded in 1982, the Department of Health announced that these were 'two isolated cases'. Consistent with Cohen's definition of isolation as a variant of interpretive denial, the event is acknowledged but is passed off as an exception (Cohen 2001: 109). Given the tremendous spread of HIV that followed, this is a position that would have been hard to maintain for an extended period of time. Moreover, it is entirely possible that at least initially, the virus did appear to be confined to homosexuals. And so, in the early years of the epidemic, whilst most infections were latent and the spread of HIV went largely unrecorded, policy makers relied heavily on *isolation* to assure the (white) public that it was not in any form of immediate danger. What makes this a probable case of official denial is that government continued to use rhetorical devices resembling *isolation* even after it became quite clear that the epidemic had become a heterosexual one and was no longer limited to a few homosexuals. Instead government actions and statements then seemed to suggest that HIV was limited to the black population. In the context of apartheid, this argument helped to set the basis for a policy of inaction that, as we note in Chapter 4, largely characterised South Africa's early response to the epidemic.

'Technically, it is illegal to spread HIV'

When officials use legal discourse to deny their responsibility it is known as *legalism* (Cohen 2001: 107). Using an entirely warped rationale and often quoting domestic or international law, officials would then argue that they could not have committed the alleged act (or that the act could not have happened at all) because it is, as they have demonstrated, against the law to do so (Cohen 2001: 108). Although the South African government did not resort to *legalism* in this way exactly, the apartheid government did find another way to make the law work in its favour – by passing a series of AIDS-related legislation that was meant regulate the spread of HIV (see Chapter 4). There is some resemblance between this use of the law and Cohen's definition of *legalism*.

The first suspected case of *legalism* goes back to 1983 when the apartheid government introduced the *Human Tissue Act*. By excluding particularly homosexual men from becoming blood donors, the act was an effort to 'legislate away' the problem of homosexuals contaminating the blood pool (as the test for HIV only became available in 1985). However, it also further cemented the idea that homosexuals are the main carriers of AIDS.

On 30 October 1987 the government enacted another two pieces of legislation aimed specifically at smothering the AIDS issue. The first, an amendment to the *Public Health Act* (63 of 1977), sought to make AIDS a notifiable disease. Any HIV-positive persons could now be placed into quarantine by order of the Minister of Health. It also allowed public service agencies to refuse services to HIV-positive individuals. This could be taken as far as refusing an HIV-positive pupil access to schooling. The second act was issued by the Ministry of Home Affairs as an amendment to the *Admission of Persons to the Republic Regulation Act* of 1987. In short, it entitled immigration officers to subject foreigners to an HIV test. If the immigrant tested positive, he or she would subsequently be declared a 'prohibited person'. Whilst this would not necessarily force the prohibited person to leave the country, the Minister of Foreign Affairs could elect to deport the HIV-positive individual. However, this move was strongly contested by the Chamber of Mines, as many of their workers were foreign immigrants. As an alternative, the Chamber offered to treat, educate and counsel the infected workers. The government agreed and no HIV-positive miner still capable of working was deported. The services offered by the Chamber of Mines – treatment, counselling and education – are fundamental services that ideally the government should have implemented.

Still, growing panic over the increased risk posed by HIV-positive foreigners motivated government to subject applicants for work permits to compulsory HIV tests if they came from countries classified by the WHO as 'high-risk'. HIV and AIDS were subsequently added to the list of conditions that barred immigrants from successfully applying for a work permit. Homosexuality, prostitution and intravenous drug use had already been criminalised and therefore did not require any more efforts at legislation.

Collectively these laws virtually criminalised the spread of HIV. Instead of engaging in prevention and treatment programmes for the general public, the South African government chose to relieve itself of that responsibility by simply legislating the issue away. Consistent with interpretive denial, this allowed government to redefine the AIDS problem to suit their own terms. It created the impression that law-abiding citizens were not at risk and therefore excused the government from responding more proactively. Importantly, it also entrenched a number of other pejorative messages around the epidemic and PWAs. Many of these messages also appear to exhibit elements of Cohen's construction of interpretive denial.

'Foreigners are spreading AIDS'

Legislation aimed at HIV-positive foreigners also reinforced the idea that HIV was spread predominantly by migrants from 'other' African countries. In addition to resembling *legalism*, this is also another very likely case of interpretive official denial – arguing 'what is happening is really something else' (Cohen 2001: 105). At a time when government could have acknowledged that AIDS had become a heterosexual issue that put the majority of the population at risk and therefore required large-scale response, it instead created a scapegoat and argued that HIV is spread mainly by foreigners. This made the apparent route of response fairly simple – stop foreigners from entering the country and spreading HIV.

'AIDS affects black people more than white people'

Constructing HIV and AIDS as a problem that concerns 'the other' appears to be a recurring theme in the apartheid government's response to the epidemic. When the government eventually launched its first HIV and AIDS campaign in 1988, campaign material appeared to convey two very different sets of messages. As was not unusual at the time, South Africa's first campaign to address AIDS was racially segregated (Furlong and Ball 2005: 130). However, messages tailored for the black audience were considerably more grave and urgent than those contained in the advertisements designed for white viewers. The 'black version' of these AIDS education advertisements featured images of a coffin and a funeral. The 'white version' on the other hand, starred a man called Kevin and told his story of promiscuity, partially through graffiti. Kevin's AIDS death was communicated very discreetly along with a vague cautioning against sleeping around. It appeared that in addition to raising awareness of AIDS, these campaigns carried another message: AIDS affected black people more than white ones (Grundlingh 2001: 138).

A survey conducted by the advertising agency that produced the campaign showed that although the advertisements created greater AIDS awareness amongst white South Africans, 89 per cent of them believed it was not necessary to change their behaviour. Only 30 per cent of the black audience felt they had no reason to change their behaviour (Grundlingh 2001: 138). This campaign, as a reflection of government's attitude towards the epidemic at the time, corresponds with Cohen's definition of interpretive official denial. The apartheid government did acknowledge the AIDS problem but again went on to give its own interpretation of the situation, namely that that HIV and AIDS pose a considerably greater threat to black South Africans than whites.

'AIDS is a social, personal issue that is out of the government's hands...'

When governments assign responsibility to forces beyond their control like psychopaths, vigilantes or mercenaries, it is considered as *denial of responsibility* – another variation of interpretive denial (Cohen 2001: 109). Although not as dramatic as allegations of vigilantism or madness, the apartheid government's repeated efforts at positioning the AIDS problem within the private, individual realm can be considered an attempt at *denying responsibility*.

Initially, when AIDS appeared to be a largely homosexual affliction, Dr Coen Slabber, Director General of the Department of Health, explained that because homosexuality was not accepted by the majority of the population and particularly not by the ruling Afrikaner elite, advocating universal condom use would be problematic (Grundlingh 2001: 126). Clearly the apartheid government considered AIDS to be the personal concern of people who should not be engaging in (unnatural) sex in the first place. By framing AIDS as a problem limited to social deviants, government claimed they had no further responsibility to them.

Around 1988, when overwhelming evidence attested to AIDS having become a mostly heterosexual disease, the government was forced to alter its position – which thus far had consisted largely of stigmatising and blaming the gay population. But their tune changed only slightly as they continued to blame individuals for their 'reprehensible' behaviour. Government's focus now shifted away from incriminating homosexual behaviour specifically to condemning sexual behaviour in general (Grundlingh 2001: 127–8). Their new scapegoat became a rather vaguely defined sexual promiscuity: having more than one sexual partner ('sleeping around') and any other form of sexual exploration that did not occur within the confines of marriage. Making this the new target of taboo was easily achieved in a conservative, prudish society. In so doing government made the issue of sexual transmission of HIV a matter of narrowly defined morals and principles. Their redefinition of the AIDS problem still quite clearly restricted it to the private realm – where it remained conveniently far removed from the government's jurisdiction and sphere of responsibility. Dr Slabber now called it a social and behavioural problem of the community (Grundlingh 2001: 128).

In 1990 the newly appointed Minister of Health, Dr Rina Venter, declared that the 'problem of AIDS is that it is not primarily a medical problem. It relates to social behaviour. You can't legislate against sexual behaviour' (quoted in Grundlingh 2001: 128). Remarkably, Venter's statement uses one form of denial, *denial of responsibility*, to justify why officials were not reverting to another form of denial, *legalism*, by legislating against issues. This points to a deeply entrenched rhetoric of denial that prevented policy makers from even considering any alternative strategies that would require acknowledging the general threat posed by the epidemic. Ironically of course, the apartheid government had been rather adept at legislating against sexual behaviour, quite contrary to Venter's statement.

'AIDS is spread (exclusively) through high-risk behaviour'

The apartheid government's continual emphasis on promiscuous sexual behaviour seemed to suggest that it is what you do, not how you do it, that gets you infected (being homosexual/having multiple partners, rather than having unprotected sex). As AIDS initially appeared to be confined to the fringes of society the HI virus was already heavily stigmatised when it made its debut in the country. When it became clear that HIV had become a heterosexual problem it was no longer blamed on morally deviant groups, but rather on morally deviant behaviour. By warning against the dangers of promiscuous behaviour government continued to frame HIV as a consequence of high-risk behaviour, rather than a result of unprotected sex. This conception of the problem meant that the only viable counter-measure to the epidemic was not education and promoting safer (protected) sex, but rather monogamy, faithfulness and abstinence. In addition to further stigmatising HIV-positive persons by branding them as sexual deviants, it created the impression that by leading an officially sanctioned lifestyle that complies with specific moral codes, it is possible to insulate oneself entirely from contracting HIV.

Whilst abstinence and faithfulness are widely acknowledged ways of minimising the risk of contracting HIV, by themselves they are by no means a comprehensive response to the epidemic. Here government's resorting to interpretive official denial created the impression that the problem has never been HIV or AIDS, but instead people's promiscuous behaviour. Moreover, their stubborn focus on high-risk behaviour obscured the fact that HIV was above all a medical condition (and not purely a societal, behavioural one) that at least in part required a medical, scientific response. This made it easy to focus on blaming the carriers of the virus, rather than on finding biomedical solutions to the virus itself. Again, government rhetoric resonates with Cohen's definition of interpretive denial.

'Virodene is the answer. The Medicines Control Council is the problem'

A number of instances of interpretive official denial may also have been present in post-apartheid government's rhetoric. On 22 January 1997 Cabinet erupted in spontaneous applause – South Africa had found a cure for AIDS! Or so they were led to believe as a small group of researchers from the University of Pretoria presented them with what was purported to be a panacea that they believed was not only effective and fast-working, but also cost a fraction of the ARVs that were available at the time. The miracle cure, Virodene, seemed not only to hold the key to end suffering in Africa, but also offered officials the opportunity to make some serious money. But this African rags-to-riches story was not to be. Instead, the story of Virodene unfolded more like a soap opera with a plot thick with deceit, betrayal, coercion and corruption – and this narrative appeared to have been woven together by interpretive official denial.

Initially, the story of Virodene seemed to be another fortuitous accident of science, likened perhaps to Alexander Fleming's unintentional discovery of penicillin. When Olga Visser and Dirk du Plessis discovered the 'anti-viral properties' of Virodene, they were not engaged in AIDS research. Visser and Du Plessis were attempting to freeze organs and then revive them for transplant when they noticed that one of the solutions that they were using had anti-viral properties (Myburgh 2007).[2] It later transpired that Virodene was in fact an anti-freeze solution (dimethylformamide: DMF).

The presentation of Virodene to Cabinet by Visser and her husband Ziggy together with Du Plessis and Carl Landhauer almost instantly secured the team a R3.7 million government research grant. Although the Medicines Control Council (MCC) warned that testing should be halted until they deemed Virodene fit for human consumption, the Health Minister, Nkosazana Zuma (then one of the wives of current South African President Jacob Zuma), seemed alarmingly unperturbed by protocol (Schneider and Stein 2001: 728). In 1996 a pilot yielded no conclusive results on the efficacy of the drug. By this point it had already been established that Virodene was in fact an industrial solvent and that it was toxic even in low doses. It had also been shown to cause liver damage.[3] Meanwhile the Vissers were

2 The scientists also claimed that their attemps to freeze and revive organs were successful. However, no other scientists has since been able to replicate the results (Myburgh 2007).

3 A joint report by the University of Pretoria and the Gauteng Health Department showed beyond all reasonable doubt that Virodene was not only ineffective but harmful to patients (Myburgh 2007).

illicitly providing Virodene to AIDS patients, claiming that they had the Health Minister's secret approval (Myburgh 2007).

The MCC's continued rejection of Virodene on the grounds of toxicity and inefficacy meant that it eventually had to face the wrath of the Health Minister. Arguing that the MCC was denying patients the 'possibility of mercy treatment' the Minister undertook a dramatic 'restructuring' of the MCC (Nattrass 2007: 43). This included the forced removal of MCC Chairman, Peter Folb, the registrar, Johann Schlebusch and the Deputy registrar, Christel Bruckner. They were replaced with political appointees. Effectively the MMC had been disbanded. Much to the Minister's dismay, however, even the 'new MCC' refused to approve Virodene and by 1999 it eventually faded from the agenda. However, testing was moved out of the country and went underground where it continued.

The Virodene saga exhibits strong characteristics of interpretive official denial. Whilst the MCC was attempting to protect the public from the potentially damaging effects of Virodene, policy makers reframed the issue in their favour and argued instead that the MCC was the real villain for denying the world this miracle cure. Put simply, government argued 'what is happening is really something else' (Cohen 2001: 105). In addition to duping the public and presenting them with a false truth (and false hopes), critics have argued that in their dogged pursuit to push the approval of Virodene the government went beyond its normal realm of authority and interfered in science – something it was by no means qualified to do. At the time there was also speculation in the media that ANC officials were influenced by the potential profits that they could have pocketed from the development and sales of Virodene. This casts further doubt on the motives of the government members that were implicated in the scandal.

'AZT and Nevirapine are toxic'

Government's insistence that ARVs are toxic (outlined in Chapters 5 and 6) – when a plethora of medical research and healthy human beings suggested otherwise – is another likely case of interpretive official denial. In 1998 the government announced that it would not be making Azidothymidine (AZT) available to HIV-positive pregnant women to limit the vertical, mother-to-child transmission (MTCT) of HIV. Initially government cited financial constraints, arguing that it was not cost-effective to purchase these drugs. However, this stance was soon thwarted when it became apparent that a) preventing MTCT would in the long run be more economically beneficial than allowing infection to spread unchecked and b) the Department of Health was actually under-spending its budget. Faced with this evidence the health department quickly changed its tune, instead questioning the efficacy and the safety of AZT and arguing that more research was needed before it would approve the treatment. In spite of reports from the MCC and the WHO that confirmed the effectiveness and safety of the drug, Health Minister Nkosazana Zuma, continued to oppose the treatment.

Some years later the government followed a similar line of argument with Nevirapine, another drug meant to prevent MTCT, but substantially cheaper and easier to administer than AZT. Still claiming toxicity, in July 2000 the new Minister of Health, Manto Tshabalala-Msimang, declined an offer from the manufacturer BoeringerIngelheim to provide the drug free of charge for five years for use in MTCTP programmes (Nattrass 2007: 62–3). When the South African Constitutional Court demanded government rollout of Nevirapine in July 2002, the Health Minister lamented that the court was forcing her to 'poison' her people (Nattrass 2007: 99). Two years later, at the 15th International AIDS Conference in Bangkok, the Minister was still making statements regarding the prohibitive toxicity of Nevirapine.

By arguing that AIDS drugs were unaffordable when they evidently were not and then later that these drugs were toxic when they were proven not to be, key policy makers appear to have used interpretive official denial to warp the issue of MTCTP into something it was clearly not. Government did have sufficient funds to provide the relevant drugs for MTCTP and these drugs were beyond any doubt effective. At a time when the real focus should have been on acquiring and rolling out treatment, policy makers diverted the attention by debating the affordability and efficacy of treatment. The real atrocity in this matter, however, is not simply that the government quite likely were resorting to denial. MTCTP is not only a means of AIDS *treatment*; it is also a method to *prevent* the transmission of HIV from a mother to her unborn child. Whilst government preferred to engage in heated debate around the science of AIDS, unborn children were unnecessarily infected with HIV.

'Anti-retroviral therapies do not cure AIDS, vitamins and vegetables do'

South African official's preference for vitamins and diet to treat AIDS, rather than medication is likely to have been a similar case of interpretive denial. Although there is a strong case to be made for the importance of a balanced diet in maintaining health, presenting nutrition and supplements as a viable *alternative* to medication is highly problematic. Advocating traditional remedies and improved nutrition instead of ARVs gives the impression that HIV and AIDS are really quite harmless conditions that can be treated or avoided by making simple dietary adjustments. Essentially, the government has reframed the harm and relocated the epidemic to a 'different, less pejorative class of event' (Cohen 2001: 106). It is important to note that former Health Minister Tshabala-Msimang did not present good nutrition as complementary to ARVs, but instead she repeatedly, over many years, indicated that some vegetables could be used as a more effective, non-toxic *alternative* to ARVs.

In suggesting that AIDS can be cured or even managed with vitamins and vegetables alone, policy makers have clearly ignored scientific and medical fact. Instead, government has at times supported what Geffen (2006) calls 'pseudo-scientists' – laypeople with no real connection to the scientific or medical field who promote alternative solutions to anti-retroviral therapies. Most infamous amongst these state-supported pseudo-scientists has been Matthias Rath. A German pharmaceutical proprietor, he established himself in South Africa in 2004 and began peddling exorbitantly priced vitamins (micronutrients), claiming that they could not only help in the body's fight against AIDS but that 'with micronutrients alone, the AIDS patients could reverse the symptoms of AIDS...' (quoted in Geffen 2004: 7).

Whilst Rath should have been discounted as a quack and paid no further heed, South African key officials have made few efforts at discouraging him. On the contrary, Minister of Health Tshabalala-Msimang made several statements suggesting her support for Rath, on one occasion telling journalists that Rath's work 'complies with and compliments' government programmes (Thom 2009: 126). Rath also enjoyed support from the National Association of People Living with HIV and AIDS (NAPWA), funded mainly by the Department of Health (Thom 2009: 122).

In addition to Rath's vitamin cocktails, the Minister of Health also actively endorsed nutritional supplements that were being peddled by a retired nurse, Tine Van der Maas. Van der Maas advocated the use of lemons, olive oil, garlic and ginger to treat people with AIDS because she was not 'totally impressed with AZT' (quoted in McGregor 2009: 133). Later, Van der Maas developed a concoction called *Africa's Solution*, containing amongst other things, African potato. The Health Minister featured in the commercial for *Africa's Solution*, advocating its use to treat AIDS (NAPWA was also listed in the credits) (McGregor 2009: 140). According to Van der Maas, Tshabalala-Msimang even referred personal friends to the former nurse for AIDS-care (McGregor 2009: 134).

Health Minister Tshabalala-Msimang also added her own cocktail to this nutritional movement. At a briefing in February 2004 she announced that garlic, lemon and olive oil were 'absolutely critical' in warding off HIV infection (Faris 2004: 1).[4] President Mbeki has also been known to support this view, telling Parliament in 2004 that healthy food and clean water are all the people need. He continued by arguing that drugs cannot lead to a healthy body (Specter 2007: 35).

The situation reached its pinnacle at the 2006 AIDS conference in Toronto where the official South African stall proudly showcased garlic, lemon, beetroot and African potato. ARVs were nowhere to be seen, resulting in grave international outcry (BBC 2006: 1; Blandy 2006: 1). As Nattrass (2007: 143) points out, whilst there is no scientific evidence that these particular foods are beneficial to people with HIV or AIDS, there is evidence that some of the active ingredients of these foods may actually be harmful for HIV-positive people. African potato, for instance, has been known to lower CD4 counts and can therefore hasten the onset of AIDS.

---

4 Van der Maas has apparently gloated that Tshabalala-Msimang's affinity for garlic and lemons in the treatment of AIDS derives from Van der Maas' own success (McGregor 2009: 139).

Advocating nutrition as a substitute for medical treatment speaks strongly to Cohen's interpretive denial. Government rhetoric around this issue clearly avoided the whole truth around treatment – yes, nutrition is important but ARVs are a highly effective and proven medical means for treating AIDS. Government instead disregarded scientific evidence and constructed an alternative interpretation of the epidemic and its treatment, suggesting that nutrition was the real solution to the problem.

'AIDS is only a little problem...'

Implicit in the argument that vitamins and vegetables are more effective than ARVs is government's suggestion that the epidemic has been severely overstated. This has been a recurring theme in post-apartheid government reaction to the epidemic and correlates strongly with what Cohen (2001: 107) refers to as 'invoking *euphemism*'. Using euphemism is a form of interpretive denial that allows government to mask the true severity of an issue.

Statements by government, like Thabo Mbeki's assertions (discussed in more detail in Chapter 6) that AIDS deaths are significantly outflanked by crime, can be considered a means of euphemising the AIDS crisis. Perhaps most dramatic of these, however, has been Mbeki's statement to a *Washington Post* journalist that he 'really, honestly' did not know anyone who has died of AIDS. This came in spite of the then recent death of ANC official Peter Mokaba from a long illness – suspected to have been AIDS related (Murphy 2003). Together with Mbeki's frequent questioning of AIDS statistics, this suggests that government did not consider the epidemic to be quite as serious a threat as it was made out to be. Again this was done as a self-exculpatory mechanism excusing government from the responsibility of an appropriate, scientifically informed response.

Implicatory official denial

When officials do not contest that the event is occurring (literal denial), or if they do not offer an alternative interpretation of the event (interpretive denial), then they can still reformulate the implications that the event might have. This is known as implicatory official denial and is the third and final category of classic official denial as defined by Cohen. By invoking implicatory denial, neither the fact nor its meaning are contested. In fact, most of the main facts are admitted to, but the consequences or implications of the issue are either denied or otherwise reformulated. This form of denial is characterised by inaction, as officials are quite obviously aware of the issue, but refuse to do something about it on the premise that it does not concern them or otherwise does not affect them (Cohen 2001: 7). In effect, implicatory official denial is a tactic employed by officials to justify suffering and in so doing, to absolve them of any responsibility that might ensue.

There are a number of ways in which implicatory official denial can be executed and the intentions behind these justifications may vary. Whilst some explanations may be sincere, others can be blatant lies (Cohen 2001: 110). Still there is plenty of room for creativity. Officials could, for instance, make an appeal to higher loyalties like religion, to argue that universal values like human rights are trumped by allegiances to certain religious principles. This tactic is referred to as *righteousness*. Alternatively officials could resort to more utilitarian approaches and say that they had no other choice but to follow the course of action they did (*necessity*). Officials could also divert attention by arguing that they are the real victims. Or they could argue that the victims should be held responsible for their own suffering as they have brought it upon themselves – either because they deserved it, or because they were the instigators ('they started it') (Cohen 2001: 110). This is known as *denial of the victim*.

Officials may also draw on the particular context of an atrocity to argue that outsiders cannot fully appreciate the complexity of the situation without being intimately familiar with the backdrop against which the problem is set (*contextualisation*). Alternatively they can appeal to the *uniqueness* of a situation to argue that the particular case cannot be compared to any other. A final tactic identified by Cohen (2001: 111–12) involves comparing actions with those of others and is known as *advantageous comparisons*. Employing this argument, officials would compare their actions to the 'much more atrocious' actions of their opponents, suggestion that they present the lesser of two evils. When dealing with critics, officials could therefore point out their shortcomings or hypocrisies. Alternatively, they may invite their critics to compare them with other countries facing similar predicaments, upon which the critics will be forced to conclude that by comparison, the situation is not nearly as bad as initially perceived.

Collectively, these approaches form a formidable set of government tactics that can facilitate the evasion of responsibility and that are frequently used by governments all over. A number of actions and statements issued by the South African government show elements of such implicatory denial.

'The rest of the world is over-reacting'

In the early years of AIDS in South Africa the apartheid government is likely to have invoked a particularly interesting form of *advantageous comparison* to justify its inaction. Some time after the first AIDS deaths were recorded the Department of Health's spokesperson, Dr George Watermeyer, justified the government's slow response by arguing that in the rest of the world campaigns could have been 'too early, too heavy' (quoted in Grundlingh 2001: 127). He further argued that the sexually explicit nature of the international campaigns would have been met with resistance from South Africans. In selecting this line of argument the Department of Health argued that compared the rest of the world, South Africa's response is more sensible and realistic than the over-reacted international responses.

'Be a good Christian, and you won't get AIDS'

The oppressive moral climate during authoritarian apartheid rule was highly conducive to arguments of *righteousness*. In fact, the very premise on which the government ruled was based around ideas that any society is entitled to its own unique construction of morality (Cohen 2001: 110). Apartheid necessitated the belief that some races are superior to others, which left no room for allegiance to universal standards like human rights. This attitude permeated the apartheid government's response to the epidemic.

In the late 1980s policy makers appealed to Christian values and urged the public to restrict themselves to one partner, preferably within marriage, or even advocated complete abstinence. This approach also entailed looking down on morally deviant (un-Christian) behaviour like homosexuality, drug abuse and 'sleeping around'. This overrode the need for any further kind of intervention. Moreover, it paved the way for another kind of implicatory denial – the argument that those who contracted HIV did so as a result of their morally deviant behaviour.

'AIDS is God's punishment'

Government's initial framing of the epidemic as confined to morally deviant members of society appears to present an attempt at *denying the victim.* Arguing that AIDS can be avoided entirely through moral behaviour suggested that those who contracted HIV did so at their own peril. AIDS, at least initially, was considered 'God's punishment' or some similar act of cosmic retribution inflicted on morally deviant members of society. A reaction of this nature, however, is not unusual. Kopelman (2005: 208) has called this negative stereotyping 'the punishment theory of disease'. This idea that sick people deserve to fall ill (as they have brought it upon themselves) bears close resemblance to Cohen's conception of implicatory denial as *denial of the victim*. The apartheid government appeared to endorse this view as is evident in the legislation at the time (see Chapter 4). Homosexuality, prostitution and intravenous drug were already criminalised when the epidemic arrived in South Africa. This further encouraged the construction of these groups as no less than deserving of the wrath of AIDS.

'ARVs are just too expensive'

Signs of implicatory denial can also be found in the post-apartheid governments' actions. Officials appear to have resorted to claims of *necessity* in their arguments that ARVs were simply too expensive. The monetarisation of the South African AIDS epidemic saw government attribute their inadequate response to forces/variables that were beyond their control. These arguments were largely underlined by a broad policy shift that began in 1996 and informed the view that if AIDS did not directly affect economic growth and employment creation, the country could not afford to make it a priority. Weaving claims of necessity into their rhetoric, government could argue that they had no other choice but to refuse the provision of treatment.

In 1998, citing budget constraints and arguments around cost-effectiveness, government declared that it could not make AZT available to pregnant women to prevent the transmission of the virus to their unborn babies. This was accompanied by arguments that large pharmaceutical companies were abusing intellectual property rights in order to profit from the sale of ARVs. As a possible solution to the issue, government drafted the *Medicines Act* of 1998 that would facilitate the development of generic treatments that would be more affordable. Not surprisingly, pharmaceutical companies were uncomfortable with the that threat generic treatments posed to their profit margins. In 2001, the American Pharmaceutical Manufacturers' Association (PhrMA), representing 39 pharmaceutical companies, took the South African government to court. The government fought back, joining forces with the Treatment Action Campaign (TAC) and resisting PhrMA court action.

However, when PhrMa eventually abandoned their legal action and ARVs were significantly discounted as a result, government did not embrace the opportunity to engage in immediate rollout. Instead it quite suddenly changed its tune, arguing that ARVs were unsafe. This startling leap of logic casts significant doubt on the sincerity of the government's initial financial arguments. As government continued to oppose the provision of treatment even though it was now affordable, their initial arguments are likely to simply have been feigned claims of *necessity* as part of a wider effort to evade responsibility.

'The South African government is being extorted'

Post-apartheid policy makers have at times also argued that they, wearing an anti-colonial revolutionist or (maybe more accurately) and African nationalist hat, are the real victims of the epidemic. This tactic involved framing the epidemic as part of the ANC's anti-colonial struggle, a battle waged against 'economic and political exploitation by multinational organisations' (Wang 2008: 3). A paper circulated amongst ANC members in 2002 extensively elaborated this argument. Titled 'Castro Hlongwane, caravans, cats, gees, foot and mouth and the statistics: HIV and AIDS and the struggle for the humanisation of the African', the paper argues that 'the West's' involvement in the African AIDS epidemic is driven primarily by pharmaceutical greed (Wang 2008: 6; Butler 2005: 606). The document also suggests that AIDS is a conspiracy devised by these companies to either depopulate the African continent with its toxic ARVs or at least to extort Africans as guinea-pigs (Butler 2005: 607). It then goes on to launch a full-scale attack on all organisations of the West that are involved in the epidemic. The 'West' is a term used rather loosely, with no real distinction made between governments, multinational companies or NGOs (Wang 2008: 7).[5]

5 'Castro Hlongwane…' contains a number of narratives that can be considered a form of official denial. It is therefore discussed again (in greater detail) later in the book. For a full version of the document, see Anonymous (2002).

The arguments contained in 'Castro Hlongwane...' that allowed officials to argue that the South African government is actually the victim in the AIDS epidemic, exhibit distinct elements of implicatory denial. The real victims in this case, however, remained unacknowledged – South African citizens who were suffering needlessly at the hands of their lethargic government. This argument also put a spin on the epidemic as a whole. Detracting from the epidemic's destructive impact, the paper suggested that the real danger of AIDS was that South Africa was being extorted by ruthless Western capitalists. This not only obscured the real issue but also relocated the blame to suggest that the West is responsible for the South African epidemic – and not the government.

'Drug companies are the real crooks'

Government officials' impassioned attacks on Western pharmaceutical companies may present another form of implicatory denial. Consistent with what was identified as *condemning the condemners* (Cohen 2001: 111–12), policy makers have responded to criticism from these companies with fierce counter-accusations. South African officials have accused these 'Western' organisations of immoral conduct, suggesting that they are extorting Africans with their over-priced drugs (see for instance Butler 2005; Heywood 2004; Wang 2008). Compared to their neo-colonialist urges to exploit Africans, government's own failure to roll out treatment appears to be only a little sin. In fact, if, as some of the arguments contained in 'Castro Hlongwane...' would suggest, AIDS is merely a conspiracy devised to facilitate this exploitation, then government's failure to provide treatment is practically negligible anyway.

'The South African case is not that unique'

In their attempts to diffuse a situation and evade responsibility for an atrocity, officials may draw on the *context* and *uniqueness* of the situation in question (Cohen 2001: 111). However, in the case of AIDS such arguments may not be entirely conceited. AIDS is, in fact, unique in its extent and severity. This position is known as 'AIDS exceptionalism'.[6] Moreover, the South African situation is very different from most others, suggesting and justifying an even higher degree of exceptionalism. As Marks (2008) indicates, and as we have explored in more detail in Chapter 2, a number of factors unique to South Africa have led to the rapid and often unchecked spread of the virus.

When AIDS first made its appearance in South Africa the apartheid politics of the day enabled great complacency and 'provided almost ideal conditions' for the spread of the virus (Youde 2007: 74). The white general population felt

6 UN Special Envoy for AIDS in Africa, Stephen Lewis, has for instance recently supported the notion of AIDS exceptionalism, arguing that it facilitates an aggressive and necessary response to the epidemic (Alcorn 2009).

unthreatened as it appeared that the epidemic was limited to homosexual white men, migrant miners and other 'promiscuous' African immigrants. The black population on the other hand discarded AIDS as a white man's disease. These views meant that the epidemic grew unchecked for most of the apartheid years.

At least two other relatively unique factors have contributed to the momentum of the South African epidemic (Marks 2008). The first is the migrant labour system in which men were forced to live in single-sex hostels far away from home. This resulted in the creation of unusually vast sexual networks. The second factor is the culture of violence and sexual abuse in South Africa, which again dramatically increases the spread of HIV.

Mbeki in particular has grappled with issues of *uniqueness* and *contextualisation*. However, in his case this has consisted mostly of questioning the tenets of AIDS exceptionalism, arguing for instance that statistics of HIV incidence are 'hysterical estimates' (Mbeki and Leon 2000) or stating that he did not know anyone who has died of AIDS (Murphy 2003).

The South African epidemic is in fact unique in its context as well as its magnitude. It truly is an exceptional situation that requires a response of exceptional intensity. Here Cohen's conceptualisation of *uniqueness* and *contextualisation* as mechanisms of interpretive official denial would need to be inverted in order to accommodate the unique context and intensity of the South African epidemic. In the South African case, claims of uniqueness and attempts to contextualise the epidemic would be entirely justified. Contesting the clearly exceptional nature of the epidemic then becomes denial by the same token that arguing exceptionalism in the case of an unexceptional event would. From this vantage point, Mbeki's doubts about the uniqueness of the South African situation and his attempts at downplaying the extent of the epidemic show strong characteristics of implicatory official denial.

Given the truly exceptional nature of the AIDS epidemic (and the South African epidemic in particular), in this case it is more the questioning of the uniqueness of the epidemic rather than appeals to it, which resembles implicatory official denial.

Conclusion

South African governments have on a number of occasions employed rhetoric that exhibited elements of classic official denial as defined by Cohen. Table 7.1 summarises the instances of classic official denial that have been discussed in this chapter.

Denial can be more subtle and nuanced than the cases we have discussed here. Typically denial of this nature occurs in two forms: counter-offensive attacks levelled at critics, or partial acknowledgement of wrongdoing without the redeeming feature of corrective action. The following chapter investigates instances where South African governments appear to have resorted to counter-offensive denial or partial acknowledgement.

Table 7.1 Summary of possible instances of Classic Official Denial

CLASSIC OFFICIAL DENIAL

Type of Denial	Official Rhetoric		Estimated Period
Literal Official Denial	AIDS only kills homosexuals, commercial sex workers and intravenous drug users.		1982–85
	AIDS is a black disease.		1985–90
	AIDS is not the biggest killer, crime and poverty are.		2000–01
	…and besides, AIDS is not caused by HIV.		2000
Interpretive Official Denial	Isolation.	Only a few homosexuals/ prostitutes/drug users are affected.	1982–83
	Legalism.	The spread of HIV is outlawed.	1983–87
		Foreigners are spreading AIDS.	Mid-1980s
	AIDS affects black people more than white people.		1988
	Denying responsibility.	It is out of the government's hands. This is a social, personal issue.	1982–89
	AIDS is spread through high-risk behaviour.		1982–88
	Virodene is the answer. The MCC is the problem.		1996–97
	AZT and Nevirapine are toxic.		1998
	Anti-retroviral therapies don't cure AIDS. Vitamins and vegetables do.		2004–06
	Euphemism.	AIDS is only a little problem…	2000
Implicatory Official Denial	The rest of the world is over-reacting.		1982–85
	Righteousness.	Be a good Christian and you won't get AIDS.	Late-1980s
	Denial of the victim.	AIDS is God's punishment.	Late-1980s
	Necessity.	ARVs are just too expensive.	1996–98
	Denial of the victim.	The South African government is being extorted.	2002
	Advantageous comparison.	Drug companies are to blame.	2002
	Claims of contextualisation and uniqueness.	The South African case is not that unique.	2000–04

Chapter 8
Counter-offensive Denial and Partial Acknowledgement

Introduction

In dealing with accounts and accusations of wrongdoing, officials often reach a point where the tactics of classic official denial no longer provide a sufficient cover or excuse for inaction. Victims and critical observers can act as powerful pressure groups that present governments with evidence that is hard to explain away or ignore. At this point officials may resort to more subtle approaches that are even more deeply couched in rhetoric and spin. Here Cohen's typology distinguishes between two further forms of official denial. The first is an attempt to subvert critics who are pointing out officials' wrongdoings and is known as *counter-offensive denial*. The second has to do with the antithesis of denial – acknowledgement. When denial is no longer an option, officials may consider acknowledging *some* of the accusations. However, this is just a *partial* acknowledgement whilst much of the facts are omitted. This usually does not give way to any action beyond that.

These strategies are common for democracies. The nature of authoritarian regimes means that they are seldom confronted by the media, civil society or the international community who might force them to abandon the arguments contained in classic official denial. Democratic governments on the other hand are more likely to use *counter-offensive denial* and *partial acknowledgement*. This chapter explores the many possible cases in which these strategies may have been invoked by the South African government in their response to the AIDS epidemic.

Counter-offensive denial

The increased transparency brought about by improvements in communication technology means that modern governments often find themselves at the receiving end of public onslaught from humanitarian organisations or other governments. When presented with well-planned arguments, written reports and documents, eyewitness accounts or statistics, officials in denial have little recourse but to retaliate with accusations of their own. Unable to engage in outright denial in the presence of an abundance of evidence, governments instead resort to a tactic described as *counter-offensive denial* in order to subvert the accusers.

This is commonly done by attacking the integrity of the accuser. Officials would then discount the allegations in their entirety as lies, propaganda, ideology, disinformation or prejudice. Their arguments are bolstered by efforts at discrediting the source of criticism. This can include an attack on the critics' source of financing, or the political affiliations of their informants, fieldworkers or board members. Officials could also argue that the timing of the report or attack is 'politically motivated' (Cohen 2001: 112). Internal critics are commonly labelled 'treacherous, unpatriotic or irresponsible' (Cohen 2001: 112).

A number of incidences, most of them recent, have exhibited elements of counter-offensive on behalf of the South African government.

'Racists!'

South African government officials have on a number of occasions, accused their detractors of being racist. As theses retorts were meant to discredit critics, rather than argue issues, these statements are by definition a form of counter-offensive attack. The earliest instance of racist counter-offensive attacks we have identified were made during the *Sarafina II* scandal in 1996. As part of an effort to inform and educate the public on issues of HIV and AIDS, the Department of Health commissioned playwright Mbogeni Ngema to produce an educational musical about HIV and AIDS. However, a number of controversies tainted the production from the start and in the end, *Sarafina II* never made it to the stage (see Chapter 5 for the full story).

Criticism came from the media, opposition parties and civil society – most prominently AIDS activists. Accusations directed towards the Department of Health and specifically the Minister of Health, Nkosazana Zuma, dealt with three main concerns. The first was related to the cost of the production. With a budget of R14.27 million, *Sarafina II* demanded a significant portion of the heath department's overall AIDS budget. Secondly, critics pointed out that the correct tendering processes were not followed and that Ngema's appointment was fast-tracked, without the proper procedures being followed. Thirdly, critics have argued that the play's message was ineffective and inappropriate.

Health Minister Zuma did not receive these accusations well. Instead of arguing issues she chose to respond by hurling counter-attacks at the media and opposition parties, accusing them of being racist. Zuma went as far as to suggest that criticism was a result of the tender being awarded to a 'black man' (Marais 2000: 33).

The following year, the Health Minister was making similar remarks, this time in response to criticism directed at the Virodene scandal. Critics lambasted the Department of Health and minister Zuma in particular, for unashamedly pushing a drug that was unsafe for human testing and most likely ineffective on the whole. Again criticism from both the official opposition in Parliament as well as the media was met with accusations of racism. This time the minister accused the opposition of wanting black people to die.

Thabo Mbeki has also resorted to accusations of racism in remarks that were clearly counter-offensive in nature. However, his onslaughts have been considerably more urbane than those of Health Minister Zuma. Mbeki's arguments have often been backward-looking with frequent historical references to the oppression of the black race. This tactic became known as 'playing the race card' – a particularly fitting label as it alludes both to the strategic, political aspect of alleging racism as well as to the fact that it is not a reflexive response but rather part of a more tactical approach.[1]

In April 2000, in a letter to world leaders, Mbeki spoke about his concern that the mainstream scientific consensus was forcing into 'scientific quarantine' those scientists with alternative views on HIV and AIDS. He likened this marginalisation of dissidents to the approaches of the 'apartheid tyranny' and conjured images of heretics being 'burnt at the stake' and 'books burnt and their authors immolated' (Mbeki 2000). Whilst the references to racism in his letter were rather limited, as Mbeki drew on a wider imagery of persecution and tyranny, the President's next counter-offensive attack required no reading between the lines. In a series of letters exchanged between Mbeki and Tony Leon, the leader of the official opposition, the Democratic Alliance, the accusations were considerably more direct. Leon had levelled serious criticism at Mbeki, urging him to provide ARVs to rape victims. Mbeki's response was long-winded, furnished with carefully selected, fragmented and misleadingly decontextualised quotes from scientific documents. In summary, his arguments suggested that HIV cannot be transmitted through rape (Mbeki and Leon 2000). His letter contained a number of rather unambiguously counter-offensive, racist attacks. He claimed that rape figures were manufactured and deliberately inflated by 'those who seem so determined to project a negative image' of South Africa. He then turned to accusations of racism, alleging that a number of people adhere to the belief that most black men are HIV-positive and that rape is endemic to African society. Mbeki also called HIV incidence figures 'hysterical estimates'. He then labelled Leon's demands that GlaxoWellcome sell discounted AZT in South Africa as 'deeply offensive and contemptuous' (Mbeki and Leon 2000).

The following year, in a strange rant at Fort Hare University in October 2001, Mbeki again resorted to counter-offensive measures that involved accusations of racism. These allegations were made in an address delivered by Mbeki at the inaugural ZK Matthews memorial lecture. This time Mbeki's references to HIV and AIDS were implied rather than explicit. Nonetheless, he devotes five paragraphs to discussing the way in which Westerners have continued to portray Africans as beings of a lower order that are unable to curb their passions and subject themselves to reason. He further argues that the West has constructed

---

1 The South African cartoonist Zapiro popularised this idea when he drew Mbeki and DA leader Tony Leon, sitting across the table from each other, playing a card game. Both politicians have placed their cards on the table. Leon's cards spell the words: A-I-D-S Sc-ie-nc-e whilst Mbeki's cards simply spell R-A-C-E. A speech bubble shows Mbeki triumphantly declaring: 'Trump!' (first published in *The Sowetan*, 16 August 2000, but referenced here as Zapiro 2005).

Africans' inability to tame their sexual urges as the main cause for the rampant spread of disease, particularly HIV and AIDS. Whilst this level of clarity and intent is inferred from his speech, the following extract amply demonstrates that drawing such conclusions are not in the least radical or assumptive:

> Convinced that we are but natural-born, promiscuous carries of germs, unique in the world, they proclaim that our continent is doomed to an inevitable mortal end because of our unconquerable devotion to the sin of lust (Mbeki 2001).

This theme of African sexuality pervades Mbeki's rhetoric, surfacing again in Parliament in October 2004 when he insisted that questions raised by MPs concerning matters of HIV and rape were racist. He argued that these kind of comments accused Africans and South Africans of being 'lazy, liars, foul-smelling, diseased, corrupt, violent, amoral, sexually depraved, animalistic, savage – and rapist' (quoted in Stephen 2009: 162).

Mbeki's references to apartheid and colonial oppression as well as the Western construction of the African as savage evolved into a complex narrative of dehumanisation. This depiction of the West allowed Mbeki to develop a complex counter-offensive argument: that statistics were exaggerated and that the efforts made by Western NGOs and pharmaceutical companies were driven by self-interest and thus simply a continuation of colonial oppression. The next section deals with this issue in further detail.

Western villains: Neo-colonial humiliation and dehumanisation

Some of the fiercest and most eloquently argued cases of counter-offensive denial have come in the form of anti-colonial sentiment as expressed by the Mbeki governments and in particular by Thabo Mbeki himself. These attacks have been predominantly structured around issues of colonial oppression and neo-colonial exploitation and effectively enabled Mbeki to bring the integrity of the West into question. As Gevisser (2007: 745) so aptly put it, 'Mbeki had an acute understanding of how colonial discourse had long rendered Africa the dark "other" and now read AIDS through this prism'. This was done by employing a counter-offensive argument that firstly accused the West of constructing Africans as savage which robs them of their dignity and secondly accused the West of exploiting Africans. The West, he argued, exaggerated their depiction of the African AIDS epidemic in order to profit from the sales of treatment. In his logic Mbeki thus transferred much of the blame for the epidemic to the developed world. In so doing he not only attempted to absolve himself and his government from responsibility for the epidemic, but also to discredit his biggest detractors and render their criticism redundant.

Arguably the most prominent and perhaps most peculiar embodiment of this anti-colonial, anti-Western sentiment is contained in the document mentioned earlier that was circulated amongst ANC members in 2002, titled 'Castro

Hlongwane, caravans, cats, geese, foot and mouth and statistics: HIV and AIDS and the struggle for the humanisation of the African'.[2] The identity of the author is not revealed in the document, however, the possibilities have been narrowed down to two.

According to Sitze (2004: 768) rumours are rife that prominent ANC official Peter Mokaba penned the monograph. Mokaba died of a lung condition only months after the document was made public. His death was widely rumoured to be linked to a long AIDS illness. On the other hand, in Mbeki's biography, Gevisser (2007: 736) argues that the variety of the sources quoted in the document has led many to conclude that Mbeki might be the secret author of the monograph. To further substantiate his suspicions, Mbeki has confessed to Gevisser that the document is a true reflection of his own views. Moreover, whilst Gevisser was writing Mbeki's biography, Mbeki sent him an updated version of the document that was nearly twice as long as the original and contained quotes as recent as August 2006.

Whilst disregarded by some, others have given the monograph considerable reflection. And when considered in the context of Cohen's typology, 'Castro Hlongwane…' reveals a strong counter-offensive narrative that sheds valuable light on motives underlying government inaction and official denial (see Table 8.1). Furthermore, Sitze (2004) has read the document against a background of the Washington Consensus and what he calls 'global apartheid' whilst Wang (2008) has used it to gain a deeper understanding of Mbeki's denial as set in the wider context of the post-colonial struggle. Both authors offer interesting insights, which will be raised in the next chapter as part of an effort to uncover possible motives for official denial.

The document's essence can be summarised into a simple battle between the 'omnipotent apparatus' and the African. This battle is set against a backdrop of continued oppression, exploitation and humiliation by the 'omnipotent apparatus' of the African.

Couching its argument in the broader notion that Africa continues to be subjected to Western prejudice, stereotyping and exploitation, 'Castro Hlongwane…' to some extent justifies governments' inaction by arguing that the West, with its constructions of the African AIDS epidemic, is attempting to humiliate the African and undermine its integrity. Simply put, the document could be interpreted to say that because the West has ill intentions, it cannot be trusted and therefore its assessments of the epidemic and advice on how it should be treated should not be paid any heed. Moreover, the document offers a justification for the Mbeki government's position on ARVs: since they are developed by Western pharmaceuticals that have ill intentions, they can neither be effective nor necessary. Furthermore, acquiring these drugs would therefore constitute the surrender of the African continent to perpetual exploitation and humiliation.

---

2 For the full text of the document, see Virusmyth (2002).

Table 8.1 Summary of key arguments in 'Castro Hlongwane...'

The Omnipotent Apparatus (OA)	The African
'Narrow-mindedly' subscribes to the scientific, orthodox definitions of HIV and AIDS.	Challenges scientific consensus.
'Believes' that HIV causes AIDS.	Rejects the 'hypothesis' that AIDS is caused by one virus.
Forces this mainstream definition upon the African and considers those who challenge it, heretics.	Argues that AIDS (or immune deficiency in general) is caused by many illnesses, most of them the result of poverty.
Argues that AIDS is the biggest challenge facing the African continent and responsible for the largest number of deaths.	Argues instead that poverty is Africa's biggest challenge and largest cause of death and that the OA is denying this.
Has vested financial and political interests in propagating the HIV and AIDS 'hypothesis'.	Is being forced to submit to this hypothesis (and consequent exploitation) to qualify for aid.
In propagating this 'hypothesis', the OA relies on colonial depictions of the African as savage and sexually untamed.	The African is humiliated through subjection to this portrayal as sexually insatiable and rapist.
Ultimately is peddling ARVs only as a means to exploit the African and therefore continue colonial oppression.	Continues to be exploited, humiliated and oppressed – and above all, is being subjected to treatment that is ineffective.

The TAC: Traitors and conspiracists

Organisations calling for the rollout of ARVs have been particularly menacing to government. Armed with medical research and statistical evidence, they exerted enough pressure on officials to affect a court order that forced government to provide ARVs (see Chapter 5 for more). It is not surprising then that government responded to this pressure with numerous counter-offensive assaults. As South Africa's largest civil society organisation campaigning on HIV and AIDS, the Treatment Action Campaign (TAC), bore the brunt of numerous counter-offensive assaults from government.

The TAC was established in December 1998 with the initial intention to transform the National Association of People Living with HIV and AIDS (NAPWA). The latter was the brainchild of co-operative efforts between the ANC and HIV and AIDS NGOs, established in the early 1990s. However, the organisation was generally considered to be lacking clout, direction and reach and the TAC wanted to turn it into a true 'mass movement' (Achmat 2009: 199; Heywood 2004: 3). Integral to their involvement in NAPWA was the TAC's intention to reform the government's 'conservative approach to the right of access to treatment' (Heywood 2004). The TAC was founded by people who had a great deal in common with the ruling ANC. As 'comrades from the anti-apartheid struggle' many were members of the ANC (Achmat 2009: 199). The TAC seemed to hold the potential for a productive working relationship between civil society and the government. Their partnership culminated in the successful defeat of the pharmaceutical giant, US-based Pharmaceutical Manufacturers' Association (PhrMA), in April 2001. PhrMA had taken the South African government to court over the *Medicines Act* of 1997 which would allow for the import and manufacture of cheap generic equivalents of patented AIDS medicines.

However, all hope of further co-operation were soon dashed when the relationship between the TAC and the government turned sour later in 2001. Despite PhrMa dropping the case the Minister of Health announced that the result would not sway her position on ARVs. In particular, Nevirapine (used to limit vertical MTCT) would not be made available beyond the 18 pilot sites where it was being tested. The TAC responded by taking the Ministry of Health to court. The bid was successful and half a year later, although against their will, the government was making Nevirapine available (Fassin 2007: 68). More discord between the TAC and the government was soon to follow.

Towards the end of 2002 the TAC together with the Congress of South African Trade Unions (Cosatu) completed a Framework Agreement for a National Treatment Plan. In spite of the fact that the National Economic Development and Labour Council (NEDLAC) had agreed to the plan, the government refused to support it. The TAC responded with a formidable disobedience campaign. On 14 February 2003 some 15,000 people marched to Parliament to launch the campaign. The protest action included further demonstrations, interruption of speeches and a charge levelled against the then Minister of Health Manto Tshabalala-Msimang and Minister of Trade and Industry Alec Erwin with culpable homicide for their failure so set ARV rollout in motion (Stephen 2009: 163).

The government frequently retaliated to pressure from the TAC with their own counter-offensive accusations, alleging treason, racism and treachery. In an ANC caucus in September 2000 Mbeki shared with his cadres the theory that the US Central Intelligence Agency (CIA) together with large drug companies were plotting against him in an effort to ultimately discredit him. The TAC, according to Mbeki, was receiving funding from these companies. The following year, at the ZK Matthews Memorial Lecture at Fort Hare University, Mbeki referred to the TAC as follows:

> ...others who consider themselves to be our leaders take to the streets carrying their placards, to demand that because we are germ carriers, and human beings of a lower order that cannot subject its passions to reason, we must perforce adopt strange opinions, to save a depraved and diseased people from perishing from self-inflicted disease (Mbeki 2001).

The TAC has often been accused of being 'anti-government'. In particular its civil disobedience campaign sparked a flurry of criticism from government officials and other affiliates. During this time the Health Minister aimed a racist attack at Mark

Heywood, co-founder of the TAC, making references to the 'white man' dishing out orders to Africans. African subservience to white males also featured in a similar attack by Christine Qunta, a close associate of Mbeki (Nattrass 2007: 115). An ANC Youth League spokesperson responded to the campaign by describing the TAC as 'a conglomeration of drug dealers who serve as marketing agents of toxic drugs' (quoted in Nattrass 2007: 115). Given the TAC's strong roots in the ANC, government's allegations correspond closely with Cohen's observation that 'insiders' are often referred to as traitors and conspiracists.

The enemy within

The government's battles with the TAC have not been the only case where groups demanding the rollout of ARVs have elicited official counter-offensive attacks. State doctors and even a Deputy Minister of Health have felt the government's wrath when they pushed for treatment rollout. Three prominent cases are discussed here.

As a result of increasing rape cases in their community, in 2000 a group of concerned citizens established the Greater Nelspruit Rape Intervention Project (GRIP). GRIP set up a care room for rape survivors in the Rob Ferreira Hospital in Nelspruit, Mpumalanga. Through discreet and efficient handling of rape cases they aspired to ease the trauma experienced by rape victims. GRIP did this by offering counselling, providing patients with a bath and a change of clothes and also handing out post-exposure prophylactic (PEP) starter kits. This was deemed a necessary step: should the victim require PEP, treatment is most effective when administered as soon as possible. As most rape cases occur and are reported after-hours when pharmacies are closed, GRIP considered the provision of a first dose of PEP vital to the success of the treatment.

However, when the Department of Health got wind that a hospital was providing ARVs, the provincial Health Minister, Sibongile Manana, launched what the then senior medical superintendent at the hospital described as a 'witch hunt'. Manana accused GRIP of 'blackmailing and undermining the government' and prohibited the further provision of PEP (quoted in Von Mollendorff 2009). GRIP was eventually disbanded. In this case, officials' efforts at framing their critics as conspirators were so pervasive that their actions led to the dissolution of a group that were doing nothing but saving the very lives the government was entrusted to protect.

A similar case occurred in rural Kwa-Zulu Natal province in 2008, but this time official rhetoric went beyond allegations of simply undermining government; the provincial minister commissioned an inquiry into racism. Manguzi Hospital came under fire when it introduced dual therapy for MTCTP without following the required protocol. There was broad consensus by that time that the single dose of Nevirapine that was given to HIV-positive mothers antenatally was not entirely sufficient to prevent newborns from becoming infected. The hospital appealed to the Department of Health to introduce WHO-approved dual therapy that involved giving birthing women an additional ARV earlier in their pregnancy. But the government turned down their request. Feeling ethically compelled, Dr Colin Pfaff procured donor funding and started women on AZT earlier in their pregnancies (Lombard 2008). The provincial Health Minister, Peggy Nkonyeni, did not take kindly to Pfaff undermining her authority and instituted disciplinary proceedings based on 'trumped-up charges of misconduct' (Heywood 2008: 17).

Following this display of 'anarchy', in a statement directed more or less at the staff of Manguzi Hospital, Nkonyeni questioned the motives of rural doctors, suggesting that they were profit seeking and did not care for their patients. Pfaff's colleague, Dr Mark Blaylock, was so incensed by the provincial minister's remark that he threw her picture in the dustbin. This gave Nkonyeni the incentive she needed to launch an investigation. The provincial Health Minister subsequently appointed a task team to investigate 'racism, ill treatment of staff and abuse of departmental facilities by Dr Blaylock and some doctors operating at…rural facilities' (quoted in Cullinan 2008). Nkonyeni also referred to the staff at Manguzi Hospital as 'people masquerading as doctors'.

The media storm has since passed and the Minister has backed off. But in their zealous pursuit of these 'racist and anarchical' doctors, government made it sufficiently clear that they were more interested in witch hunts than in saving lives. The government rhetoric that developed during the Manguzi Hospital incident brims with counter-offensive denial. Dual therapy was sorely needed and the doctors at Manguzi Hospital, far from being self-interested bigots, were simply doing what they felt compelled to do given the vacuum of official accountability. But this made government look inefficient and that was not acceptable. The only way to escape further accountability was to tarnish the reputations of the offenders. Official denial cost a remote rural hospital two excellent and compassionate doctors (Heywood 2008: 17).

Official counter-offensive attacks were not limited to government doctors. In 2007 the Deputy Minister of Health, Nozizwe Madlala-Routledge, was dismissed on familiar accounts: not following protocol. When Minister of Health Manto Tshabalala-Msimang took an extended leave of absence due to ill health, Madladla-Routledge stepped in and took a firm biomedical stand on HIV and AIDS. She challenged AIDS denialism, lobbied for ARV rollout, took a public AIDS test and referred to the epidemic as a crisis. But according to the Health Minister her Deputy was out of line. Upon her return from sick leave, Tshabablala-Msimang admonished Madladla-Routledge and urged her to withdraw from the AIDS debate. Madladla-Routledge however continued to gall her superiors with her interest in public health. When the Deputy Minister paid an apparently unauthorised visit to Frere Hospital, the neglect at which she consequently described as a 'national emergency', the government had had enough. Using accounts that she had travelled to an international AIDS vaccine conference without the President's permission, Madladla-Routledge was asked to resign; the Deputy Minister refused to do so and consequently, in early August 2007, Thabo Mbeki fired her (see Chapter 6 for more). The Deputy Minister's open dialogue about the epidemic challenged government's inaction, and their response to her criticism was to accuse her instead of corruption and defiance. This resounds clearly with Cohen's description of counter-offensive denial.

Partial acknowledgement

Democracies have reputations to maintain. Consequently their responses to accusations of inhumane activity can eventually amount to partial acknowledgement of the issue (Cohen 2001: 113). However, as Cohen (2001: 113) further indicates, this cannot be equated to complete acknowledgement, as officials usually invoke one or all of the following devices in order to avoid full responsibility.

Officials will concede to an event but also make it clear that this was an isolated incident that is entirely unsystematic and uncharacteristic of the system (and will not be repeated). This is known as *spatial isolation.* Government might also point out that what happened was in the past – *temporal containment.* In so doing, present leadership presents itself as separate from the erring former dispensation. The third device involves *self-correction* as a means to escape further criticism. The accused officials would claim that they are aware of the issue and have already taken steps to correct the situation.

According to Cohen (2001: 115), these strategies are so widely practiced that they have become part of a 'culture of denial' in which most people accept partial acknowledgement as normal government response without it evoking any suspicions of serious denial. Differentiating between a government's sincere regret and intentions to rectify an issue and merely feigning crocodile tears can be tricky. The definitive factor here is action that brings about a tangible change. Partial acknowledgment seldom goes beyond paying lip service to a problem. Many of the South African government's responses have failed to translate into real action. Most of these exhibit some form of partial acknowledgement. The most notable ones are reviewed here in a chronological manner.

Lip service: Apartheid governments' lacklustre responses

In the initial stages of the epidemic the South African government did very little to respond to HIV and AIDS. Still, the issue was on the agenda and a few steps, though insufficient and lacking enthusiasm, were taken by the government in response to the epidemic (refer to Chapter 4 for a more comprehensive account). As this seldom went beyond public declarations of their intentions to respond to the epidemic, many of these could be considered a form of *partial acknowledgement.*

Initial attempts were confined to insulating those members of society who were of 'value' to the apartheid government. This meant that government's earlier responses were comprised mostly of efforts at securing blood supply. Initially, this was achieved by enacting legislation, namely the *Human Tissues Act* (65 of 1983), which barred certain high-risk groups from donating blood, specifically homosexuals.

When the first clinical tests for HIV were made available in 1985, ensuring the safety of blood required a less stereotypical approach. At this time some funding was made available for education campaigns, research, training and counselling (Van der Vliet 2001: 153). Still, no efforts were made to address the real at-risk groups. In fact, the pre-existing morally damning attitude towards their 'socially unacceptable' behaviour meant that these groups were already legislated against and were of little further concern to white society at large.

Moreover, because the narrow definition of carrier groups initially ruled out heterosexual transmission and the apartheid government disregarded health issues in townships, squatter camps and homelands, 'black communities did not receive the attention or resources they deserved' (Grundlingh 2001: 126). Whilst authorities presented the situation as 'under control', their disregard for human rights and their narrow-minded prevention-only approach meant that the reality of the situation was both obscured and more importantly remained unaddressed in the early years of the epidemic. However, in 1988 when it became apparent that AIDS had made the transition to heterosexuals, the government began taking more tangible steps.

By the late 1980s the extent of the AIDS epidemic began to dawn on the state. In 1987 the MRC established an AIDS research unit that confirmed an increase in heterosexual transmission. At this time R1 million was set aside for AIDS (Van der Vliet 2001: 153). The white Minister of Health, Dr Willie Van Niekerk, announced that 'the disease certainly has the potential to become a major problem' (quoted in Grundlingh 2001: 127). This could be considered an attempt at *self-correction* – admitting that there is a problem and that the government is aware of it. However, the government's lethargic reaction to its own observation entrenches this realisation as a rhetorical device rather than as a indicator of real action.

The following year the Department of Health announced an alarming increase of AIDS amongst African miners and the communities close to the mining compounds. It became clear that AIDS was a growing concern and the state showed increasing awareness of the threat AIDS posed to the general population (Furlong and Ball 2005: 131). Focus now moved away from who you were (homosexual, drug user, prostitute) and instead came to rest on what you did – engaging in high-risk behaviour (Grundlingh 2001: 127). This changed emphasis could be construed as an attempt by the apartheid government to isolate the incidence of HIV infection and feign a sense of control. By suggesting that the disease was limited to what you do, officials endeavoured to isolate the issue.

By this time the white government had little choice but to begin changing its attitude and policies towards HIV and AIDS. Moreover, the changing political climate in the late 1980s meant that government had to draft more appropriate policies and retract its discriminatory legislation. During this period *partial acknowledgement* appears to have presented itself in a number of forms: for instance, in her 1990 budget speech the then Minister of Health, Dr Rina Venter, announced plans to reconstruct the health services and to redress racial inequality and segregation (Furlong and Ball 2005: 133). The Department of Health also called for increased community involvement, arguing that creating awareness was not a sufficient response. To this end it began establishing training and information counselling centres in major cities (Furlong and Ball 2005: 132). This approach was coupled with open and frequent public declarations that the fight against the spread of AIDS was 'a matter of great concern and a high priority' for the government (Grundlingh 2001: 128).

That is, at least on paper and in their speeches. However, in reality the politics of the day took priority and the issue of AIDS fell by the wayside (Grundlingh 2001: 128). It increasingly transpired that in spite of its publicised intentions to address the issue of HIV and AIDS, the state failed to back up its commitment with adequate funding. Moreover, campaigns were either racially stereotyped or their messages were widely misdirected and ineffectual (Grundlingh 2001). Also, none of these early efforts really curbed the spread of HIV (Furlong and Ball 2005: 134). This tepid response speaks strongly to *partial acknowledgement*, specifically *self-correction*. The government repeatedly conceded its awareness of the issue and broadcast its intentions of taking the necessary steps to redress it. However, in its application this response proved to be inadequate and in all likelihood was meant to be more of a diversion than a real response.

The long talk to freedom: NACOSA and the transition period

By the early 1990s the onus of the AIDS issue began to move away from the apartheid government; HIV and AIDS instead became the burden of the ANC and its partners who would soon be leading the country into a new democratic era. However, the government-in-waiting was preoccupied with the final vanquishing of the apartheid government and the pursuit of reconstruction and development. Consequently, whilst the ANC, COSATU and their affiliates were well aware of the AIDS situation, 'a coherent plan to address the disease eluded them' (Van der Vliet 2001: 159). And so, in spite of Communist Party leader Chris Hani's repeated warnings of a looming plague, the first two years of the 1990s were marked by further inaction.

However, AIDS issues did not disappear from the agenda entirely. As the country moved towards democratisation the changing political atmosphere opened a window for the redefinition of the AIDS problem – specifically as a human rights and development issue. This generated increasing interest from civil society and pressure mounted for the country's key decision makers to participate in a newly democratised dialogue on the epidemic. So in 1992 stakeholders gathered under the banner 'South Africa United against AIDS'. Working in union, members of the incumbent white government, key ANC members, trade unionists, AIDS activists and members of the medical community established the National AIDS Convention of South Africa (NACOSA). Although the ANC largely takes credit for this, the apartheid government played an instrumental role in the process (Furlong and Ball 2005: 132). This was clearly an unusual show of national unity.

The members of NACOSA developed and intended to implement a national strategy on HIV and AIDS. They dubbed it the National AIDS Plan (NAP). Of the eight drafting members, two went on to be the consecutive first Health Ministers of the new government (Van der Vliet 2001: 160). This meant that when the ANC came into power they already had a 'formidable strategy, on paper at least, for addressing HIV and AIDS' (Butler 2005: 593). However, at this stage the NAP was still only a proposal. Its true value and therefore the extent to which the government would honour its promise address the epidemic, would only really be revealed upon implementation.

Planning to fail: The implementation of the NAP

The NAP was adopted by Cabinet in 1994 and received wide acclaim both for its democratic process and comprehensive content. The plan embodied six key elements: (1) education and prevention, (2) counselling, (3) health care, (4) human rights and law reform, (5) welfare and (6) research (Marais 2000: 12). (The NAP is discussed in greater detail in Chapter 4). Whilst the plan seemed theoretically sound, upon implementation two key obstacles surfaced. In its idealism, the NAP had grossly overestimated the resources the new government would have at its disposal. It also faced resistance from the very government that helped design it. Whilst restraints on resources cannot be factored into a consideration of *partial acknowledgement*, the government's failure to implement the plan to its full potential can.

Instead of assigning it a place in the President's office, from which it was originally intended to operate for the sake of swift implementation and oversight, the NAP was delegated to the Department of Health (Butler 2005: 593; Schneider and Stein 2001: 726). This left the NAP vulnerable to further curtailment on the regional level, especially in the face of competing claims on resources and effectively marginalised AIDS issues against more urgent political pursuits (Butler 2005: 593). In spite of its failure the NAP was not amended or even scrapped and remained an ineffectual policy in place. This led Nattrass (2007: 40) to conclude that 'AIDS did not seem to be a priority in the early years of the new democracy'.

It is important to note that had the NAP been implemented successfully, it could not have been considered denial. However, once the ANC came to power AIDS did not enjoy the priority status envisioned by the NAP. These responses suggest that the government may not have intended to see its plan through with the same rigour and enthusiasm it initially espoused. When considered in this light, the establishment of the NAP could be seen as a way both of saying 'although we let the AIDS issue go unaddressed in the past, we will not let it happen again' (*temporal containment*) as well as '… we have turned a new leaf' (*self-correction*). This partial acknowledgement cost South Africa dearly. Whilst the NAP was broadly heralded as a near-perfect strategy, its bedevilled implementation meant that it failed to make significant inroads in the fight against AIDS.

That said, the NAP faced a number of challenges upon implementation that were simply unforeseen. The heated political environment of the time posed further obstacles to its success. This cannot contribute to any argument around partial acknowledgement. However, it is government's subsequent failure to take away lessons from the contested NAP and use those to work towards a more viable AIDS policy that raises suspicions of partial acknowledgement. Significantly, in the absence of a workable AIDS strategy, infection spread rampantly during this time. This meant the burden of future infection and illness was mounting at an alarming rate and would inevitably impact on future governments' response to the epidemic.

'We're working on it...'

A number of further plans were devised to succeed the NAP. None were implemented with great enthusiasm or success, again raising questions about government's true intentions in responding to the epidemic.

The first attempt at recourse came in 1997 in the form of a National Health Review. In essence the Review was a resuscitation of the original NAP that took simply to reiterating the basic undertakings of the Plan and offered little revision or reflection on the many issues of implementation the NAP had faced. Consequently, the Review failed, as the NAP did, to take the reality of the public policy environment into account. Simply echoing the optimism and idealism that characterised (and doomed) the NAP meant that the Review suffered a similar fate. The consistency of this approach with the tactic of *partial acknowledgement* soon becomes apparent. The Review offered the government a real opportunity to acknowledge the NAP's failures and redress them effectively through action. Instead the Review became a PR tool that created the illusion that the government was serious about implementing an effective AIDS policy.

The Mandela government made one final (failed) attempt at renewing its AIDS initiative. The NAP was again revised and this time was re-issued and implemented under the title of the new 'Governmental AIDS Action Plan (GAAP)'. GAAP was unveiled at an AIDS crisis summit. Already here the lack of true commitment was embarrassingly obvious. The Minister of Health showed up late and then Deputy President Mbeki considered the opening of the World Athletics meeting more important, making only a brief appearance at the summit.

A month later great efforts were made to officially introduce GAAP to the public. On 9 October 1998 the South African government announced its new 'Partnership Against AIDS' during a highly publicised television broadcast. President Mandela was meant to introduce this latest overhaul of the NAP to the public. However, he pulled out at the last minute and Deputy President Mbeki was forced to stand in. Lacking the charisma of Mandela, Mbeki was awkward, unalluring and came across oddly mechanised as he read off a teleprompter. This sent a clear message to the public that most of the noise made about AIDS was just that – noise, with little intention of real action.

Officials' preference for partial acknowledgement over real action appears to have persisted under Mbeki's new leadership. In 2000 the government launched the *HIV and AIDS and STD Strategic Plan for South Africa: 2000–2005*. The new plan espoused a multi-sectored commitment to fighting the epidemic that sought to involve a broad base of stakeholders (Butler 2005: 595). The Strategic Plan called for the creation of a number of institutional structures that would be tasked with implementing the plan. These included the South African National AIDS Council (SANAC), the interdepartmental committee on AIDS (IDC), a collection of the Health Ministers of each of the nine provinces (MinMECs), a committee of the provincial heads of health (PHRC), provincial AIDS councils (PACs) and a forum comprised of the directors of health. It also restated the importance of the Department of Health's HIV, AIDS and STD Directorate.

However, the Strategic Plan was in many ways yet another derivative iteration of the NAP. Key decision makers had decided to rather review existing goals and objectives than draw up a new plan from scratch. The Strategic Plan was commended for its inclusive approach. However, as in the case of the NAP, it suffered a similar crisis of implementation. Moreover, in its implementation it became harrowingly clear that the government again was not committed to implementing the policy it had formulated. The composition of SANAC is one such an example. It was meant to be comprised of 16 members of government, 17 members were to be selected from civil society and the Deputy President would act as chairperson. However, upon its establishment government appointed all members – most of them from the government, with hardly any scientists, clinicians or pharmaceutical companies present. It had also neglected to include the AIDS consortium: a network of around 200 AIDS NGOs. Policy on the regional level showed a similar lack of implementation. Processes were so cumbersome and structures were so inefficient that in the first year that the National Integrated Plan was implemented on a regional level, the regions managed to spend only around a third of its budget.

The drawn-out spectacle involving the NAP and its two successors (GAAP and the Strategic Plan) is evidence of government's lack of intent and/or ability to follow through on the policies it formulated. This tendency to say (and put onto paper) one thing and then do something entirely different (or not do anything at all) resounds strongly with *partial acknowledgement*.

ARV rollout drags on

A similar proclivity for partial acknowledgement is found when looking more specifically at the rollout of ARVs, in particular HAART. The South African government's resistance to make ARVs publicly available is well known and widely publicised and has been a recurring theme throughout this book. Following their long-winded battle with civil society (particularly with the TAC), the Department of Health eventually conceded legal defeat and in November 2003 drew up an Operational Plan for rollout. However, the reluctance of the Health Minister to follow through on the undertakings of the Operational Plan made government action again appear to be a case of partial acknowledgement. After the publication of the Operational Plan drug procurement continued to be torturously slow and treatment guidelines were only made available in September 2004. The programme was only fully launched between 2005 and 2006 (Nattrass 2007: 128–31).

Introducing dual therapy to prevent MTCT was an equally painfully slow process. In 2005 the WHO recommended that dual therapy be used to reduce the likelihood of a mother transmitting HIV to her unborn child. The following year the medical community and civil society began pushing for the government's single-dose regimen to be adapted accordingly. However, it was only in 2008, after a great deal of prodding and not without a fair share of controversy and counter-offensive allegations that the Department of Health finally released new MTCTP guidelines in February 2008. Again, failure to follow through on prior commitments resulted from appeared to have been government's continued official denial.

Looking forward: The NSP

Towards 2007 things were looking hopeful. Possibly driven by the embarrassment of the Toronto AIDS conference (at which the South African stall's proudest exhibit appeared to be its denial of the science of AIDS), in 2006 Cabinet finally engaged in discussion of the AIDS crisis with a new-founded sense of urgency. The reigns were tightened on the controversial Health Minister, Manto Tshabalala-Msimang, and the Deputy President was tasked with the restructuring of SANAC. Civil society, including the TAC and AIDS Law Project (ALP) were key to the newly improved SANAC, which went on to draft the new *National Strategic Plan for HIV and AIDS 2007–2011*.

However, this newfound display of solidarity between government and civil society was not without upheavals. The review of the previous Strategic Plan was hasty and lacking in scientific method. Also, even though the Minister of Health was on sick leave, she still successfully inconvenienced SANAC through her influence on health officials. Nonetheless, SANAC's drafting of the latest NSP was a milestone and a turning point for South Africa's epidemic. The final draft was presented at a consultative meeting where it was made open for scrutiny from a variety of stakeholders and appropriate amendments were made (Heywood 2006: 17–18). However, again Health Minister Tshabalala-Msimang was opposed to the NSP and refused to champion it (Heywood 2008: 14); in doing so the Minister seemed to be at odds with even her own officials.

Conclusion

Counter-offensive denial and partial acknowledgement are subtler types of official denial. As a result they are harder to identify and argue convincingly. However, as this chapter has demonstrated there have been a significant number of incidents that can safely be considered counter-offensive denial and partial acknowledgement. These are outlined in Table 8.2.

Chapters 7 and 8 have shown that South African governments are likely to have repeatedly resorted to official denial when dealing with the HIV and AIDS epidemic. A number of recurring themes have come to light that may shed more clarity on the underlying motives of official denial. Whilst it is difficult to prove government denial beyond a doubt, this investigation of South African official denial does provide a number of clues about government's actions over the last 28 years. The following chapter is dedicated to making explicit the politics underpinning government denial.

Table 8.2 Examples of nuanced forms of denial

Type of Denial	Official Rhetoric		Estimated Time
Counter-Offensive Denial	Racists!		1996–2004
	Western Villains: Neo-colonialism and dehumanisation.		2002–06
	The TAC: Traitors and Conspiracists.		2000–02
	The enemy within (racists and anarchists).		2000/1, 2008
Partial Acknowledgement	Self-correction.	AIDS has the potential to become a serious problem.	1987
	Spatial isolation.	Having AIDS is about what you do.	1988
	Self-correction.	Health services will be reconstructed to redress racial inequalities.	1990
		AIDS is a matter of great concern and high priority: Calls for community involvement, establishing counselling and information centres (with little effect).	Early 1990s
	Combinations of temporal containment and self-correction ('AIDS mismanagement is a thing of the past, this is a new, highly effective plan…').	South Africa unites against AIDS: AIDS becomes a human rights issue and NACOSA is established.	1992
		The National AIDS Plan.	1994
		The National Health Review: Revising the NAP.	1997
		Governmental AIDS Action Plan (GAAP).	1998
		HIV and AIDS and STD Strategic Plan for South Africa: 2000–2005.	2000–05
		Operational Plan to roll out ARVs.	2003

Chapter 9
The Politics of Denial

Introduction

The application of Cohen's typology of denial to a specific history of government actions and inactions reveals a number of inconsistencies and possible loopholes in 'proving' official denial. Accusations of government denial are always more easily made with the advantage of hindsight. It is also virtually impossible to know the true intentions or sincerity of a government, or to accurately gauge what reality this denial should be measured against. This is especially challenging when dealing with governments as a collection of individuals. In the South African case some members of government may have been quite lucid about the state of the epidemic and have true intentions of targeting HIV infections.

This suggests that there are a number of other forces and dynamics at play (beyond individual motivations) that could eventually culminate in official inaction and possible instances of outright official denial. These are inherently tied into political considerations and strategies. These politics of denial are complex and could vary from ostensibly rational financial arguments to more emotive reasons relating to issues of culture and race. This chapter explores the politics of denial in order to achieve a better appreciation of the circumstances that might create situations where official denial becomes the preferred official response.

Motives for the denial of AIDS

Cohen's typology is an interesting tool for investigating the theory of denial we have outlined in Chapter 3, but on its own it cannot offer any explanations as to what the underlying political motivations for the South African government's resorting to denial may have been. Nonetheless this framework has provided a sound basis for further exploration of these factors and through application of the typology much of the speculation on the reasons for denial have been exposed.

Didier Fassin (2006: 70–72) has identified three common themes that have significantly influenced AIDS controversies in post-apartheid South Africa. These are issues of *national identity*, issues of *race* and issues relating to *conspiracy theory*. He argues that most HIV and AIDS controversies have been framed in terms of one of these narratives. Virodene, for instance, was considered an African cure – something that would significantly bolster the South African *national identity*. In this book we acknowledge Fassin's themes but we propose an extended set of possible motivations for political denial – eight in all, which are outlined in the following pages.

Ignorance-induced denial

It is likely that one of the initial drivers for government denial of AIDS was an overall lack of knowledge and understanding of the issue. Although it cannot be used to justify the apartheid government's discriminatory response, initially AIDS appeared to be limited to the isolated fringes of South African society. With little means of measuring its prevalence and a limited understanding of the disease and how it was spread, it might have genuinely seemed as though AIDS did not pose a serious threat to society as a whole. This left limited incentive for the government to respond.

This ignorance appeared to continue for the most of the 1980s. As Grundlingh (2001: 135) notes, the apartheid government's efforts in the late 1980s to legislate against foreigners bringing AIDS into the country, together with efforts to deport migrants that were already ill, can be considered an indication that 'there was, even in high government circles, not a clear understanding of what the disease was all about or what the appropriate actions should be'.

Issues of national identity: Enforcing apartheid and facilitating reconciliation and development

The onset of the AIDS epidemic quite unfortunately coincided with significant political instability. The apartheid government was on the verge of collapse and AIDS seemed like a minor threat by comparison. Afterwards, during the transition to democracy, South African policy makers were understandably preoccupied with maintaining the peace and bringing about reconstruction and development. This meant that at least for the first decade AIDS took the backseat to politics. As Van der Vliet (2001: 155) has put it, 'the superheated political climate between 1984 and 1994 ensured that people of all ideological persuasions interpreted, manipulated, or ignored [the AIDS issue] to suit their own political agenda'. In the same vein, Furlong and Ball (2005: 128) argue that whilst the transition to democracy hampered the De Klerk government's response to AIDS, the need to transform the state after dependence distracted the Mandela government's efforts. Fostering national identity and ensuring political stability (both for the apartheid governments and the new democratic dispensations) took precedence.

However, failing to respond adequately to HIV and AIDS could have been more than simply a matter of neglect. It may have been a strategic, political decision, taken in pursuit of nation-building goals. By way of example, recall the apartheid government's initial response to the epidemic: stigmatising and ostracising vulnerable groups and then largely ignoring the issue for the next three years; this could have been a consequence of their wider policy of apartheid (Grundlingh 2001: 126). As the apartheid government took interest almost exclusively in the general white public and AIDS seemed to be limited to marginal groups that the government already considered 'expendable' (homosexuals, commercial sex workers, intravenous drug users and black migrants) there was virtually no incentive for action. This attitude may have also underpinned the government's disinterest in addressing HIV and AIDS in black townships and homelands (areas that were far removed from the white public). Furlong and Ball (2005: 127) have called this a 'logical' response by the apartheid government.

As apartheid rule drew to a close, AIDS issues continued to be pushed to the wayside, in spite of the matter appearing repeatedly on ANC and COSATU agendas and being emphasised from public platforms, particularly by Chris Hani (Van der Vliet 2001: 158). Again, political goals may have deliberately been favoured above addressing the emerging epidemic. It is widely thought that AIDS could deliberately have been downplayed by the ANC to ease the re-integration of exiles and political refugees who were facing fierce stigmatisation. The apartheid government spread rumours in townships that returning exiles were carriers of this new plague (Van der Vliet 2001: 159). In all likelihood this was not entirely untrue – many exiles came from countries where the epidemic had reached severe proportions, like Zambia and Uganda. This meant that many of the returning ANC members were ill (Gevisser 2007: 730). Consequently, for the ANC, AIDS became a highly sensitive and deeply personal issue. The epidemic struck South Africa at the time that the ANC was gearing up for power. The coincidence of the epidemic with the return of the ANC seemed to raise the awkward question whether the ANC may have brought both liberation and AIDS (Gevisser 2007: 730). Moreover, at the time AIDS was simply not a priority and instead issues like housing, unemployment, poverty and violence received most of the attention (Grundlingh 2001: 128; Van der Vliet 2001: 159). South African policy makers at time may therefore have made a conscious, political decision to deny or otherwise disavow HIV and AIDS in favour of what appeared to be more urgent and immediate concerns.

Defensive denial: Trying to save face

Marais (2005: 18) has speculated that some of the denial resorted to by the new ANC government may have stemmed from the fact that most of the new government's critics chose to attack the ANC on the domain of HIV and AIDS (coupled with issues of crime and violence). During the *Sarafina II* scandal, the Virodene saga and arguments about the toxicity of AZT, critics and the media repeatedly exposed the government's inability to get AIDS governance right.

At the time there was also the rise of a formidable civil society that would be the cause of many headaches for the new government. The TAC had become immensely adept at challenging the government, to the extent that it could successfully take the government to court to demand it do its duty. In its campaigning the TAC has successfully rallied support from a number of organisations to exert pressure on the government on the grounds that it was 'disregarding the lives of its citizens' (Marais 2005: 19).

During the civil disobedience campaign the TAC launched a form of low-intensity warfare that went beyond their original pacifist forms of demonstration. The tactics employed in the disobedience campaign were 'barely legal' and included provocation, epitomised by the TAC charging Minister of Health Manto Tshabalala-Msimang and Minister of Trade and Industry Alec Erwin with genocide. Fassin (2007: 113) proposes that the TAC's civil disobedience campaign employed the same strategies that the liberation movement resorted to in their fight against apartheid. This effectively equated Mbeki's government and its politics to that of the reviled champions of Afrikaner nationalism and the apartheid regime.

The government was clearly deeply offended. At his infamous outburst at Fort Hare University in 2001 Mbeki accused the TAC of considering themselves self proclaimed leaders that considered Africans to be of a lower order who cannot restrain their sexual appetites and therefore require foreign intervention to prevent them from succumbing to their passions and consequently dying of AIDS (Marais 2005: 19; Streek and Forrest 2001).

It is likely that these criticisms provoked official denial as a means to restore the government's reputation after suffering public humiliation on this scale. Denial in this sense could have been a political tactic to divert attention from this sensitive issue.

Dealing with a legacy of insubordination, humiliation and Western domination

Denial could also have been a political tool invoked to restore dignity of another kind. Black Africans and black South Africans in particular share an extensive history of suffering and insubordination. Their continued marginalisation, first as a result of colonialism and then apartheid, has entrenched generations of black South Africans in a state of chronic poverty, making them acutely vulnerable to disease. As a result, HIV and AIDS have disproportionately affected the black South African population. AIDS therefore is not just one more hardship to add to their already desperate plight; it is also deeply symbolic of the continued oppression and marginalisation of black South Africans.

Against the backdrop of this history of insubordination and exploitation, Western AIDS activists' and (particularly white) scientists' involvement in Africa and South Africa especially, present a startling paradox (Wang 2008: 6). In a sense Mbeki's scepticism of Western science and his fascination with AIDS denialism become 'understandable' (Wang 2008: 4), if not excusable. Moreover, in recent history AIDS and its science have been closely linked to apartheid efforts at eliminating the black race through biological warfare (Fassin 2007: 161). Butler (2005) similarly suggests that apartheid and its racist science, together with the discourse of *uhuru* have left powerful and rational policy makers of the new South African democracy inherently suspicious of any supposedly benevolent Western biomedical paradigm. Instead these policy makers would be predisposed to an ameliorative/nationalist paradigm. Schneider and Fassin (2002: 49) have also argued that the apartheid legacy has provided an incentive for Mbeki to defy conventional (Western) science in favour of an African solution to the problem of AIDS.

This makes AIDS a deeply political issue and yet again sets the stage for politically motivated official denial. It also sheds new light on Mbeki's determination to argue that poverty is the underlying cause of most deaths in South Africa. This further complicates issues of accountability, for if poverty leads to AIDS and the West is largely responsible for African poverty, then African leaders cannot solely carry the blame for the African AIDS epidemic (or so the African nationalist logic goes).

This strong association between AIDS and Western oppression and exploitation makes it a useful narrative tool that facilitates the expression of a number of injustices and indignations inflicted on Africans. Primary amongst these is racism. In South Africa the peaceful transition to independence required reserve and restraint. Black South Africans were never truly allowed to express their outrage at apartheid and colonialism and had to suffer these indignities in silence. Denialism – particularly its rejection of mainstream, Western science and arguments that poverty causes AIDS – can provide a channel through which some of this pent-up resentment is finally articulated. In this sense denial could have been part of a political effort to argue that the reality of racism and apartheid are still too fresh to be consigned to the past (Marais 2005: 18). It could be argued that the application of denial in this case has allowed for AIDS to become a perverse kind of political catharsis for the oppressions of colonialism and apartheid.

The strong association between AIDS and Western oppression also has serious implications for (South) African development. Wang (2008: 15) has argued that this wedges denial of AIDS between 'the post-colonial struggle for state sovereignty' and 'the economic apparatus of international development'. In Wang's assessment, Africa's second liberation requires a complete independence of foreign aid. The continued involvement of the West in South Africa's AIDS epidemic is therefore deeply symbolic of Africa's continued dependence on its former oppressors. This makes AIDS a severely humiliating experience and as the notorious 'Castro Hlongwane…' document has suggested, dehumanises the African (Virusmyth 2002). In this view, AIDS denial is inextricably linked to a defiance of neoliberalism and neocolonialism in the interest of African development and the pursuit of true independence and human dignity.

This ameliorative/nationalist paradigm (as formulated by Butler 2005) has most strongly been expressed in the pursuit of an 'African Renaissance'. The evolving rhetoric of denial as expressed by members of the ANC and Thabo Mbeki has therefore become a tool in the wider pursuit of political goals associated with Afro-nationalism (Marais 2005: 18). Simply put, AIDS denial, with the manner in which it so blatantly shows two middle fingers to the West, fits in closely with the pursuits of the African Renaissance: it denounces racism and colonialism, rejects Western definitions and interpretations of Africa and instead argues that Africa has the right to define itself on its own terms (Marais 2005: 19).

In this sense it is possible that governmental AIDS denial has at times been part of a political effort to pursue an African Renaissance that would finally liberate (South) Africa from Western domination.

Institutional incapacity

It is also possible that resorting to a rhetoric of denial was more a matter of necessity than strategy. Successive South African governments may have been facing an issue that is simply beyond their capacity. As Poku and Whiteside (2006: 252) suggest, the lethargy that underlines governments' reactions to HIV and AIDS is often the result of far more urgent issues taking precedence over AIDS (consider the plethora of other issues plaguing the continent: political and economic instability, poverty, hunger, lack of infrastructure and so on). Denial then becomes a necessary way of 'coping', as dealing with all of these issues simultaneously is virtually impossible (Barnett and Whiteside 2006: 6).

South African governments' use of this rhetoric of blame and denial could present a similar way of 'coping' by simply pushing AIDS-issues to the wayside. Mary Crewe pointed out this type of incapacity already in 1998 when the government announced its 'New Partnership Against AIDS' and called for support from the public sector – perhaps not just because it desired broad-based involvement but because it was unable to manage on its own (quoted in Van der Vliet 2001: 166).

Gevisser (2006: 732) on the other hand, has proposed a type of mental or emotional incapacity. The ANC laboured ceaselessly to bring about the liberation of black South Africans. The struggle for freedom demanded the lives and dignity of many South Africans. Once the ANC had come to power, they faced the challenge of establishing a new government that would function effectively and efficiently as well as to build a nation of tolerance and peace from a long history and cultures of hate and racial difference. AIDS presents a third challenge that demands the sacrifice of more lives and dignity; this must be addressed simultaneously with the urgent tasks of reconstruction and development. This could be 'one bridge too far' for the ANC (Gevisser 2006: 732). Official denial could therefore be a response to a general fatigue amongst policy makers, as well as to a sense that the challenges they are facing are endless.

The epidemic itself

There are also those scholars who consider the unique characteristics of the AIDS epidemic in themselves as a cause for political denial. Here a great deal of insight can be gained from the study of long-wave events.

Barnett (2006: 301) attributes complacency to the crisis to three factors: firstly, scepticism towards the magnitude of the event in the face of little concrete evidence, secondly, a general inability to redress the issue and finally because of the lack of urgency brought upon by the epidemic's slow, creeping nature.

Whiteside et al. (2004: 133) call this a lack of 'lived experience' of the epidemic. As governments only deal with time horizons as long as their terms of office and as the effects of AIDS are often only visible over periods of longer than four or five years, this means that to many governments the epidemic simply does not seem urgent enough to enjoy priority status. Denial could therefore be a political strategy to avoid action and instead pass the burden on to the next administration. Our preceding discussion of the epidemic as a long-wave sheds more light on this argument (see Chapter 3).

Moreover, accounts of the epidemic are usually closely tied to apocalyptic descriptions of its devastating impact. This, together with the fact that there is no vaccine for HIV and no cure for AIDS, creates a situation in which denial is the only alternative to a state of utter desperation and despair (Sitze 2004: 771).

Financially motivated denial

During the Mandela administration the South African government has resorted to monetary arguments to justify their decision not to provide AZT for MTCTP. They took this argument to its fullest potential, using this rationale to draw up legislation that would facilitate parallel importation of generic drugs. In this particular case, however, conceptualising the issue in financial terms proved to be a faulty argument on a number of levels. All of these provide insight into possible motives for official denial.

Initially the government argued that the cost of testing all pregnant women, providing counselling, baby formula and administering the actual drug would amount to too much and simply be unaffordable. However, leaving argues about morality aside, actuarial studies on the cost-effectiveness of ARV provision soon proved that government would actually save resources through the implementation of MTCTP programmes, as treating (often orphaned) children with HIV and AIDS is a much more costly affair (not to mention the lost potential of human life). In addition to these assessments it surfaced that at the time when the government employed its misguided monetary argument it was actually under-spending its AIDS budget. It was when this evidence was uncovered that government changed its argument, insisting instead that ARVs were toxic and ineffective.

These instances of denial could have been motivated by a more sinister consideration: greed. An investigation by Myburgh (2007) suggests that senior leaders of the ANC had vested financial stakes in a locally developed AIDS treatment – Virodene (discussed in detail in Chapter 5). Myburgh's research suggests that some South African policy makers stood to gain large sums of money from the sale of Virodene. Moreover, some of the funds for the initial development of the drug had come directly from the Thabo Mbeki's office. The official denial employed in efforts to stall the implementation of ARVs (through arguments of affordability, toxicity and effectiveness) could therefore have been part of an attempt to push for the sale of Virodene instead.

That said, providing anti-retroviral treatment remains an expensive undertaking. Whilst governments may have sufficient funding in their coffers to cover such expenses, providing treatment may imply reducing expenses on other issues. For instance, the money used to provide one person with a cocktail of ARVs for one month could otherwise be used to put 17 children in school for that some period (Fourie 2006: 40). As is the case with issues of poverty, matters of nation-building, institutional incapacity or a history of colonial oppression, motives for denial are often tied strongly to real events and issues that provide great insight into the motives for officials' denialist behaviours.

Issues of culture, race and blame

This final set of possible explanations takes on a triad of very sensitive, often highly personal issues. Cultural and racial biases may foster cultures of denial that pervade society and are therefore also manifest in the actions of government officials. Culture is the lens through which people interpret actions and events. In South Africa, cultural traditions and practices have significantly influenced interpretations of the epidemic and have in many instances propagated situations of denial.

In the early years of the epidemic, black and white culture contributed to denial in very different manners. At the time the wider context of apartheid significantly informed these cultures. On the one hand, as Grundlingh (2001: 145) explains, the apartheid government effectively 'trained' white South Africans to classify people in terms of race. Labelling blacks as *inferior* and *other* made it possible for whites to allocate the blame for HIV and AIDS principally to blacks. Amongst whites, this lead to the association of physical illness of blacks not with their marginalisation and the squalid conditions that apartheid forced them into, but rather with their sinful and morally deviant, sexually primitive behaviour (Grundlingh 2001: 148).

The prevailing conservative Afrikaans Calvinist culture of the time further entrenched denial of HIV and AIDS amongst white South Africans. Their prudish attitude meant that these Afrikaners strongly opposed any conversations about sex in public – or at schools in particular (Grundlingh 2001: 149). They approached the issue with an 'abstinence only' attitude that suggested that HIV was the consequence of immoral behaviour rather than unprotected sex.

On the other hand, for black South Africans apartheid fostered an entirely different cultural take on HIV and AIDS. A constant suspicion of the government meant that HIV and AIDS were simply interpreted as another device constructed by the apartheid government to kill off the black population or, less brutally, to discourage population growth (Fassin 2007: 161–8). The growing culture of violence meant that to black youth AIDS became just another threat to their wellbeing. The threat posed by AIDS seemed almost negligible compared to the threat of persecution, imprisonment and death. As Van der Vliet (2001: 159) put it, for them it was a case of 'eat, drink and be merry, for tomorrow we die!'.

Traditional African culture has also introduced further incentives for denial. In an intriguing ethnographic investigation Rödlach (2006) grouped together issues of witchcraft, imperialist conspiracy and HIV and AIDS in an effort to better understand how and why some African cultures respond to HIV and AIDS the way they do. Rödlach (2006: 110) emphasises the importance of understanding the causes and origins of a disease in traditional healing. If plausible narrative for illness cannot be provided, traditional healers often resort to blaming particular people within the community. In the absence of effective health care and ARVs, narratives of witchcraft and sorcery have become a means of coping with otherwise unthinkably desperate issues.

South African culture features further idiosyncrasies that facilitate the spread of HIV. Often these hit cultural nerves and could further foster climates of denial. Amongst these is the issue of multiple concurrent sexual partners. In some South African cultures polygamy is a widely accepted practice. Most prominent amongst advocates of multiple partners is South Africa's new President, Jacob Zuma, who already has close to 20 children and married his most recent wife (decades his junior) in January 2010.[1] As a whole, having multiple, overlapping partnerships – often over longer periods of time (as opposed to one-night stands) – is a frequently occurring practice in South Africa.[2] Moreover, women in compromised economic situations are also likely to engage in transactional sex (coitus in exchange for goods like food, clothes or money) with older men (Leclerc-Madlala 2003). Often these relationships also span over longer terms, increasing exposure to HIV and other STIs (Dunkle et al. 2004). Adding to sensitivities regarding these issues is the taboo of criticising matters deemed as 'culture' – multiple concurrent partnerships (MCPs), particularly when they are intergenerational and crafted as cultural practice, are very difficult to address. Of course this is exacerbated by issues of race; MCPs and intergenerational and transactional sex have come to be associated more strongly with the black population.

The sexual manner in which HIV is spread and the cultural issues associated with sex make this is very personal and sensitive issue. For some policy makers it has been easier to avoid the issue than face this awkwardness and address it.[3] Unfortunately, decisions made on such personal grounds can have very serious political repercussions.

---

1 See for instance Brulliard's (2009) article: 'Which Mrs. Zuma Will Be South Africa's First Lady?'.

2 Studies by Morris and Kretzschmar (1997); Parker et al. (2007) as well as Pettifor et al. (2005) provide further insight into these issues.

3 For instance, Nelson Mandela, preferred for his Deputy (Mbeki) to deal with issues of HIV and AIDS, as it was deemed 'improper' for an elder statesman to address issues regarding sex (Nattrass 2007: 40).

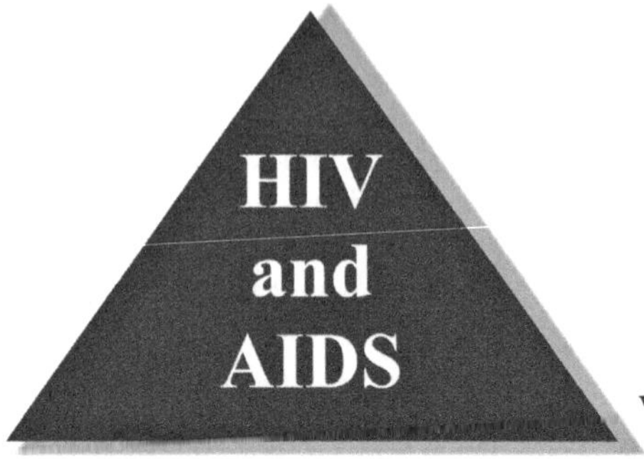

Figure 9.1 The atrocity triangle
Source: Cohen (2001).

Victim, bystander or perpetrator?

As a final reflection on the politics of denial it is useful to recall Cohen's so-called 'atrocity triangle' that we discussed in Chapter 3 (Cohen 2001: 15). The atrocity triangle (Figure 9.1) is a reminder that denial can be perpetrated from all three angles of a wrongdoing. It can be the victim who suffers the atrocity who chooses to deny this experience. Or the perpetrator can deny committing the wrongdoing. Lastly, the bystanders can deny witnessing the atrocity – or indeed that it happened at all. Bystanders can be either immediate, external or entire states can be bystanders of unacceptable acts (Cohen 2001: 15).

South African policy makers in all likelihood have been implicated in all three corners of the atrocity triangle. For one, by failing to take appropriate action they can be seen as bystanders. Secondly, through their inaction they have caused unnecessary suffering to be inflicted on the very people they have been entrusted to look after, effectively making them complicit in the atrocity. Finally, as individuals, subject to the same virus their population is exposed to and by not taking appropriate action, these policy makers have turned themselves into victims of their own denial.

Conclusion

This chapter has demonstrated that official denial can be the result of a rich assortment of underlying political issues. Official denial can almost always be explained as the result of another precipitating political factor. This would suggest that official denial is seldom a symptom of a government's general lunacy (as some critics have suggested). Instead, denial can often be explained: it can, for instance, be rooted in deeply humiliating and troubling personal issues or real concerns for development. Understanding these causes of denial is a critical condition for successfully addressing official, political denial.

That said, understanding the causes for denial does not always guarantee redressing the situation, or excuse pathological behaviour. Sometimes government denial is a function of an oppressive regime. In that case, as in the case of the apartheid government's official denial, understanding the underlying political drivers of denial does provide interesting insights, but is unlikely to result in recourse.

Chapter 10
Conclusion

Successive South African governments' continued inability or unwillingness to adequately address the AIDS epidemic has led critics to suggest that these governments have been in a state of denial over the AIDS epidemic. These accusations of denial have been the loudest when levelled at the two Mbeki governments' continual questioning of the science of AIDS as well as foot dragging on treatment rollout. However, when considering the long-wave nature of the epidemic it becomes apparent that inaction has been a symptom of government's response to HIV and AIDS from the very onset of the epidemic. From this a more complex theory of denial emerges, which postulates that successive South African governments may have been in a continual state of denial over the HIV and AIDS epidemic since the first two South African AIDS deaths were recorded in 1982.

Chapters 7 and 8 presented an effort at investigating this theory of denial through the application of Stanley Cohen's typology of official denial. In order to establish to what extent this theory of denial is valid, two factors need to be assessed; they relate to intensity and consistency. First, a judgement needs to be made regarding the significance of official denial. As this book has demonstrated, instances of government denial have been present and whilst it is difficult to prove, they appear to have also been significant. Second, an evaluation must be made to establish whether these instances of denial have been frequent enough to support the accusation that several South African governments' denial has been a consistent trend. In order to achieve a general overview of the frequency with which instances of official denial have occurred, all of the instances of government denial discussed in this book are plotted on a timeline below. To provide further context, the escalating epidemic is also included in the graphic.

Figure 10.1 shows clearly that official denial (at least as defined by Cohen) has by no means been limited to Mbeki's tenure. However subtle, it is a theme that reaches back to the onset of the epidemic and punctuated every era of leadership.

Summary of main findings

We hope that this book will have generated greater awareness of official denial, as well as the ease with which it can go undetected. The analysis has also revealed the potentially devastating impact that inaction brought about by denial can have for a country and its people.

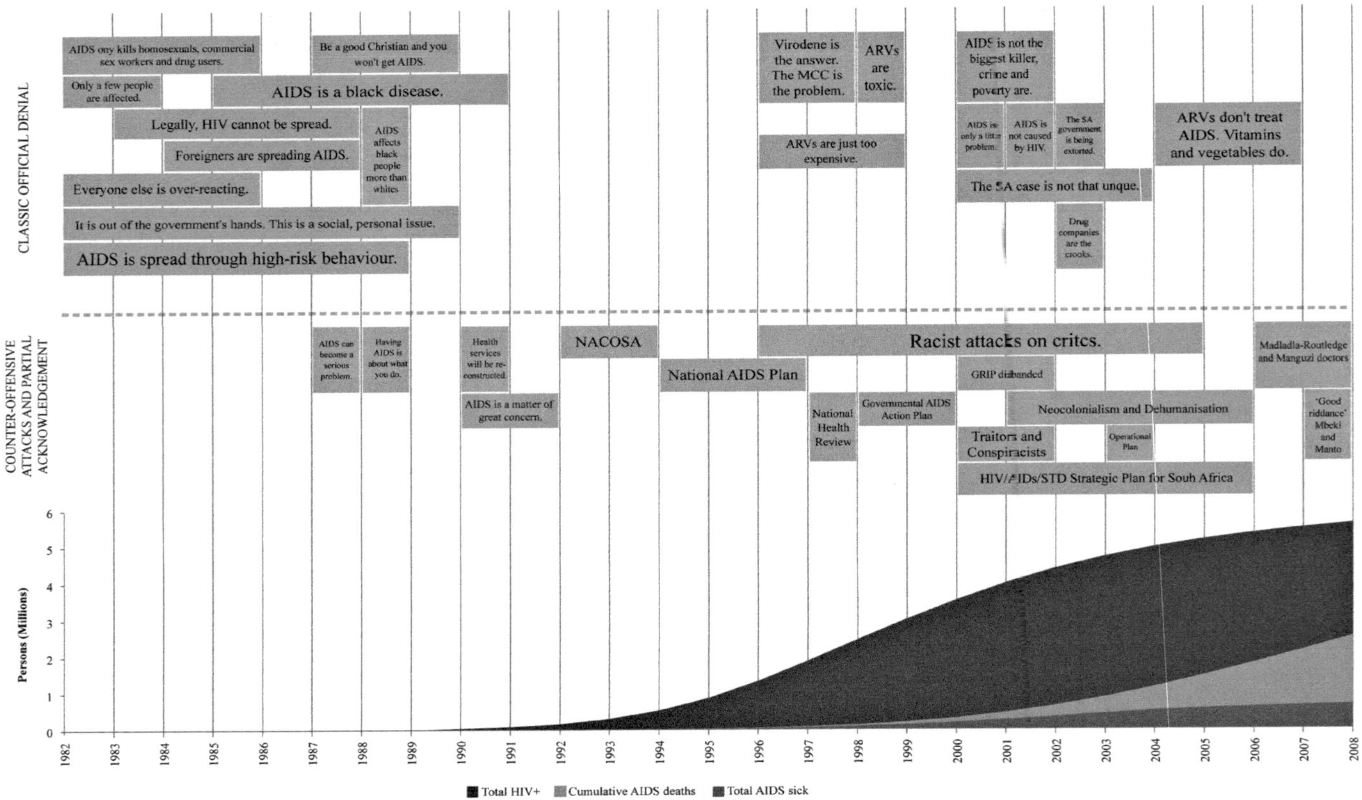

Figure 10.1 Summary of main findings

Moreover, the complexity of the HIV and AIDS epidemic has meant that this book extended beyond merely investigating this theory of denial, touching amongst others on issues of long-wave events, leadership and political motives. Our findings are outlined below.

Official denial is always political

Even when official denial is a result of the prevailing cultural climate or the personal preferences of a policy maker, the repercussions of these actions are always deeply, deeply political. In fact, official denial appears to often be assimilated into the normal government rhetoric of public relations and spin where critics and the public simply know it as 'politics'.

The blinkered pursuit of a national agenda often leads to official denial

Official denial can be motivated by any number of political factors. Often these mitigating factors can be traced back to the overall goals of the government. The various governments discussed in this book have pursued vastly different political agendas. These goals have often conspired to produce very different reasons for denial of the epidemic. They have also had implications for the types of denial that have been resorted to. In spite of their different motivations, the fevered pursuit of their agendas has caused these governments to resort to denial of some form.

The apartheid government, in its narrow-minded pursuit of the exclusive improvement of white South Africans is perhaps most glaringly guilty of this offense. Striving towards a society that is a stronghold of an exclusively defined morality and racial purity, official denial of HIV and AIDS at a time when it seemed to be limited to 'deviant' social groups was hardly a surprising response. In fact, this 'HIV and AIDS pestilence' in many ways presented a welcome vindication of the position of morally upright citizens, suggesting that: 'they have brought this upon themselves with their shameful behaviour'.

Even when the epidemic had made its transition to a heterosexual one in the late 1980s, the apartheid government found that continuing their tactic of denial still left them neatly aligned with their goals of Afrikaner nationalism. At the time it became increasingly clear that the epidemic was slowly devastating black populations, leaving white South Africans only marginally affected. This appeared to be widely and unashamedly welcomed by officials.

During the transition period, the goals of nation building and reconciliation largely trumped any issues related to HIV and AIDS. Again, this opened the door to denial of HIV and AIDS. An increased focus on human rights during that time further entrenched a lack of focus on the epidemic itself as attention was focused on those infected. In its pursuit of equality, government largely failed to pay sufficient heed to the disease itself and therefore failed to prevent further infections. Official denial at this point appeared to be more a matter of ignoring the issue in its entirety than engaging in denialist rhetoric. Because it is practically impossible to prove denial at this level, the context of the rapidly escalating epidemic must be factored into the discussion to show that a prominent and pressing issue was disavowed by the government.

Under Mbeki's rule, the pursuit of an African Renaissance, of which the restoration of Africans' dignity and intellectual enlightenment is an integral part, created further opportunities for official denial. It set the stage for the rejection of Western science and medicine and provided incentive for the creation of a narrative in which AIDS was the fault of the West almost entirely. This justified South Africa's determination to 'go it alone' in addressing the world's worst AIDS epidemic. To a large extent, Mbeki's fascination with AIDS denialism and his theories that HIV and AIDS were a plot devised by the West to extend their hold on Africa can be explained by this narrative.

The wider goal of economic development can also to some extent be considered a contributing factor in arguments that ARVs were too expensive.

A government's preferred type of denial is usually aligned with the political climate of the day

The level of transparency and civil liberties afforded to its citizens appears to bear a significant influence on the kind of denial a government may resort to. For instance, the authoritarian press model and draconian censoring legislation enforced during apartheid meant that the government could 'get away' with literal denial of the epidemic. No one could hold the apartheid government accountable or exercise any kind of leverage that could force the government into acknowledging the situation.

However, since democratisation the media, the international community and civil society have all kept a close eye on the South African government. For the large part, strategies of denial appear to have adapted accordingly to include *counter-offensive measures* and *partial acknowledgement* that allow for more subtle diversions and evasions of responsibility and accountability.

It is not just Mbeki

This book shows that although there is a great deal of uproar about Mbeki's dabbling in AIDS denialism, instances of official denial have by no means been limited to Mbeki's administrations.

It is possible that the stark contrast between truth and denial in Mbeki's contestation of AIDS *science* has finally created the necessary awareness amongst critics to spark outrage. Previous efforts at denial could simply have slipped under the radar as they were considerably more subtle. Moreover, the political climate during the apartheid era also meant that government response was insufficiently scrutinised and criticised by the media, civil society and the international community. Also, government denial at that time was commonplace and did not lead to much outcry – it was, after all, to be expected from such a tyrannical regime.

Even Nelson Mandela preferred to keep AIDS issues under the radar where they would not cause public outcry or embarrassment. When there was no way around the issue, Mandela typically devolved responsibility to his Deputy, Mbeki. And so by comparison Mbeki has been the most vociferous in this area. He for the first time drew considerable attention to issues of HIV and AIDS in South Africa – unfortunately almost entirely for the wrong reasons.

This book introduces a measure of perspective that has been greatly lacking in assessments of South African governments' responses to HIV and AIDS. Official denial has been an almost omnipresent phenomenon and whilst Mbeki's actions did receive a disproportionate deal of airtime, he and his governments have not been alone in their application the denial strategy. The real tragedy is that Thabo Mbeki probably fiercely believes his own denial script. Moreover, as we have argued earlier, Mbeki took over command of the country at a time when a great deal of latent infections began to develop into illness and death. His administrations therefore had to bear the brunt of a burden that his predecessors effectively created or at least contributed to. However, the long-wave nature of the epidemic meant that whilst he was not necessarily responsible for the state of the epidemic, Mbeki and his governments were held accountable none the less. It is likely then that this unbalanced nature of the epidemic may give way to further incentive for official denial.

Denial and blame are two sides of the same coin

Denial is generally used to escape from or divert responsibility for a particular situation. This is often achieved by blaming something or someone else. It follows that where there is denial, there usually is blame. Sometimes the converse is also true. As we have alluded to earlier, the long-wave nature of the epidemic makes this denial-blame synergy particularly complicated. When the delay between cause and effect in the AIDS epidemic is not properly accounted for, blame tends to be falsely allocated and could create situations in which denial appears to be the only way out.

Although it is hard to prove with certainty, this may have been the case with Mbeki. As is demonstrated in detail in Chapter 5, during Mbeki's term of office many latent HIV infections developed into full-blown AIDS illness and South Africa suddenly found itself firmly in the clutches of a harrowing epidemic. Add to this Mbeki and his Health Minister's denialist tendencies and it was not long before the blame for the epidemic was allocated to Mbeki and his government, when in actual fact the responsibility for inaction lies with leadership five to ten years earlier. Whilst this does not absolve any leadership from responsibility, it does offer more insight into possible causes for denial.

As leaders are ill-equipped to deal with long-wave events, they are more likely to resort to denial

This book confirms Tony Barnett's observation (outlined in Chapter 2) that because long-wave events fall outside of the normal time frames for politicians, it is extremely difficult for leaders to recognise and address them. However, we propose an addition to Barnett's observation. As mentioned in the preceding discussion of blame, long-wave events have serious implications for responsibility and accountability. The fact that effect and consequence are so far apart means that the reward for action is often located beyond the political leader's term in office. In other words, someone else will probably get the credit for former leaders' actions. This facilitates denial, as avoiding the issue might seem more effective and logical than tackling an insurmountable challenge that the politician in question will most likely never be praised for anyway.

Moreover, with long-wave events leaders also find themselves having to 'clean up someone else's mess' whilst still getting the blame for it. Again this creates situations in which denial seems to be an easy alternative.

Denial is inherently vague and volatile and therefore very hard to prove

Through the application of Cohen's typology to the South African context it has become clear that denial is a very difficult accusation to level at any government. Moreover, the more democratic and transparent the government, the harder it is to provide evidence to support such an allegation. In effect, accusations of denial have been easier to make and prove when referring to the authoritarian apartheid regime than the post-apartheid 'new' South Africa.

Accusations of denial also seem more justified when they are levelled at regimes that are generally considered to be immoral anyway (as in the case of the apartheid governments). The opposite is true for democratic regimes. Alleging that South African officials were in denial about AIDS during the transition from apartheid to democracy, for instance, simply because they did not follow through on their commitments to HIV and AIDS, may seem too harsh. During the transition period denial was barely a feature of government action. Perhaps failure to engage in effective action truly was more a case of preoccupation than actual denial. However, when viewed against the progress of the epidemic during that period, it becomes apparent that effective intervention at this point would have had a positive impact on the epidemic. Whilst denial at that time seems to have been almost negligible, the consequences of this inaction are not.

At this more subtle level, drawing conclusions of official denial may be more a function of the motives of the analyst – as denial can neither be proven nor disproven with certainty. Successfully exposing denial at this point becomes an almost impossible undertaking. It might also be possible that official denial at this level is so ingrained in government response and so refined that even though it is present, it can never be truly identified. At such a subtle level, without concrete evidence, accusations of denial will probably only provoke an official counter-response that contains only more nuanced denials that are even harder to prove. Careless accusations of denial (confusing it with ignorance, for instance), could therefore simply fan the fire, further reducing the possibility of successful intervention or action.

Those alleging denial must remain cognisant of this volatility of denial and exercise the necessary discretion. After all, rhetorical battles can only yield limited success, and in the end effectively redressing inaction or wrongdoing is considerably more important than exposing government denial for its own sake.

Areas for future study

This book has merely scratched the surface on issues relating to long-wave events, HIV and AIDS and denial. A number of areas could be investigated further.

The role of the media in the politics of denial

It could be useful to investigate the utility of Communication Theory to improve understanding of how official denial is communicated. Government denial is effectively a matter of rhetoric that is conveyed not in policy documents but in public communication, which in turn is presented to the public via the media. The media in this sense becomes a vehicle for government denial.

However, their watchdog function means that the media is also an important platform where government are held accountable and therefore the means through which their use of denial would be exposed and addressed. Often accusations of denial spark further denial by the government, effectively fuelling the fire. As Helen Schneider (quoted in Marais 2000: 34) has remarked, 'Maybe if Zuma (the Health Minister) wasn't so visibly under pressure from the *Sarafina* scandal, then perhaps it could have just slipped away and we could have got on with things'. It would be interesting to explore both the extent to which the media can assist in identifying official denial as well as its ability to address it.

Personalities vs. policies in the politics of denial

An interesting area for further investigation would be to establish the extent to which officials' personal beliefs influence their rhetoric. Gevisser (2007: 735) for instance has suggested that Mbeki's construction of his own character as a 'prophet-in-the-wilderness' has largely fuelled his affinity for the denialist position. Historically, Mbeki has been known to advocate hugely unpopular views – suggesting conversation rather than combat during the fight for independence or aligning South Africa's economy with Western market principles in spite of the widely preferred socialist approach. In both these cases, some would say that vindication came and his intellectual position was deemed triumphant. This may have caused him to favour the unconventional position in the HIV and AIDS crisis, thinking that again after great tribulations he would ultimately be proven correct.

The way forward: A scapegoat for a clean slate

There are numerous explanations for government denial. Many of these can be entirely feasible – like lack of resources, prioritising other challenges over public health, genuine ignorance and lack of knowledge and (particularly in the case of HIV and AIDS) not having the necessary foresight to plan and anticipate. We hope that this book highlights the subtleties of denial, and to point out that Thabo Mbeki alone could never be the only responsible official or the only one to have denied or disavowed the epidemic. Denial has been an ongoing symptom of government's and sometimes also society's response to the epidemic. Also, in the same way that there was official AIDS denial before Mbeki, it appears to have persisted even after he and his disastrous Minister of Health were replaced.

South Africa has entered a new phase of government response to the epidemic. The implementation of the NSP, driven by the restructured SANAC, seems to hold the promise for an end to official inaction and denial. There has been meaningful public dialogue on the devastating influence of Thabo Mbeki and Manto Tshabalala-Msimang. In an almost cathartic spirit, Mbeki and Tshabalala-Msimang have been officially acknowledged as major obstacles to implementing an effective treatment plan – the South African Young Communist League has gone as far as suggesting that the former President and Minister of Health should be charged with genocide (Letkotjolo 2009).

This new era of talking openly about the mistakes of the past could be one of two things – it may be a necessary precursor to constructive action, or (once again) it could be a way of allocating blame to the past in an effort at partial-acknowledgement, absolving present leadership from the responsibility of mopping up and moving on. After all, as Mabogoane (2008) stated shortly after Mbeki's sacking, '[a]t no stage in his almost decade-long presidency of both the party and the government did the [African National Congress] raise any objections to Mbeki's statement or actions, including his positions on HIV [and] AIDS'. Mbeki's legacy on AIDS is not his alone, and turning Thabo Mbeki into a scapegoat now is dishonest, disingenuous, and frankly too little too late. This retrospective mud-slinging and self-exculpation are also distracting from active steps towards redressing the epidemic.

One can only hope that this attempt at creating a clean slate is not a precursor to more official denial and the further evasion of responsibility, but instead that it sets the scene for a different kind of leadership that is truly willing to face a long-term crisis – and do so honestly, and with greater humility.

Bibliography

Achmat, Z. 2009. Remembering a decade of the Treatment Action Campaign. In: K. Culminan and A. Thom (eds) *The virus, vitamins and vegetables: The South African HIV/AIDS mystery*. Auckland Park: Jacana Media.

AFP. 2000. South Africa-AIDS-Mbeki: HIV 'cannot cause a syndrome'. *Agence France-Presse*, 20 September. <http://www.aegis.com/news/afp/2000/AF000968.html> accessed 29 July 2009.

Agenda. 2002. The Department of Education's life skills, sexuality and HIV and AIDS programme. *Agenda*, 53.

AIDS Analysis Africa. 1991. ANC to test its exiles for AIDS. *AIDS Analysis Africa*, 2(2).

AIDS Analysis Africa. 1994. Editorial. *AIDS Analysis Africa*, 4(6).

AIDS Analysis Africa. 1995a. Africa veers between inertia and coercion. *AIDS Analysis Africa*, 6(1).

AIDS Analysis Africa. 1995b. AZT on trial to stop mother-to-child transmission. *AIDS Analysis Africa*, 5(5).

AIDS Analysis Africa. 1999. Information, ignorance and the politicisation of AIDS. *AIDS Analysis Africa*, 9(5).

AIDS Consortium. 1993. The AIDS Consortium charter of rights on AIDS and HIV. *South African Journal on Human Rights*, 9.

AIDS Scan. 1990. International conference on health in Southern Africa releases draft statement on HIV and AIDS in Southern Africa. *AIDS Scan*, 2(2).

Ainsworth, M. 1999. Government priorities for preventing HIV and AIDS. *AIDS Analysis Africa*, 9(4).

Alcorn, K. 2009. AIDS exceptionalism a defensible concept, says Stephen Lewis. *AIDSmap.com*. <http://www.aidsmap.com/en/news/A291920E-B57E-444F-8644-E9B4E129C71F.asp> accessed 1 August 2009.

ALQ. 1999. 1999 Legislative review. *AIDS Legal Quarterly*, February.

Altman, D. 2006. Taboos and denial in government responses. *International Affairs*, 82(2).

Altman, D. 2008. State fragility, human security and HIV. In: M. Foller and H. Thorn (eds) *The politics of AIDS: Globalization, the state and civil society*. Houndmills: Palgrave Macmillan.

ANC Today. 2004. Nevirapine, drugs and African guinea pigs. *ANC Today*, 4(50).

ANC. 1994. *National Health Plan for South Africa*. Johannesburg: Shell House.

Anderson, B.A. and Pillips, H.E. 2006. *Adult mortality (age 15–64) based on death notification date in South Africa: 1997–2004*. Report No. 03-09-05. Pretoria: Statistics South Africa.

Annual survey of South African Law. 1993. Johannesburg: Juta & Co, Limited.

Anonymous. 2002. *Castro Hlongwane, caravans, cats, geese, foot and mouth and statistics: HIV/AIDS and the struggle for the humanisation of the African*. <www.virsumyth.com/aids/hiv/ancdoc.htm> accessed 10 June 2009.

Anthony, J. et al. 1995. Need for SA policy on HIV in pregnancy. *South African Medical Journal*, 85(9).

Arndt, C. and Lewis, J.D. 2000. The macro implications of HIV/AIDS in South Africa: A preliminary assessment. *Journal of South African Economics*, 68(5).

Avert, 2008. AIDS in South Africa: Treatment, transmission and the government. *Avert.org*. <www.avert/org/aidssouthafrica.htm> accessed 8 June 2008.

Avert, 2009. History of AIDS. *Avert.org*. <www.avert/org/aids-history.htm> accessed 8 June 2008.

Badcock-Walters, P. 2002. Education. In: J. Gow and C. Desmond (eds) *Impacts and interventions: The HIV and AIDS epidemic and the children of South Africa*. Pietermaritzburg: University of Natal Press.

Baeten, J.M., Celum, C. and Coates, T.J. 2009. Male circumcision and HIV risks and benefits for women. *The Lancet*, 374(9685).

Barnett, T. 2006. A long wave event. HIV/AIDS, politics, governance and security: sundering the intergenerational bond? *International Affairs*, 82(2).

Barnett, T. and Clement, C. 2005. HIV/AIDS impact: So where have we got to and where next? *Progress in Development Studies*, 5(3).

Barnett, T. and Whiteside, A. 2006. *AIDS in the twenty-first century: Disease and globalization*. 2nd edition. Houndmills: Palgrave Macmillan.

Barolsky, V. 2003. *(Over)extended: AIDS review 2003*. Pretoria: University of Pretoria.

BBC. 2002. Rape – Silent war on SA women. *BBC News*. <http://news.bbc.co.uk/2/hi/africa/1909220.stm> accessed 20 July 2009.

BBC. 2006. AIDS experts condemn SA minister. *BBC News*. <http://news.bbc.co.uk/go/pr/fr/-/2/hi/africa/5319680.stm> accessed 25 August 2008.

Beckmann, J.L. and Prinsloo, J.G. 1993. Some legal aspects of AIDS in schools and other educational institutions. *South African Journal of Education*, 13(2).

Bell, C., Devarajan, S. and Gersbach, H. 2003. *The long-run economic costs of AIDS: Theory and an application to South Africa*. Washington, DC: World Bank.

Berger, J. 2001. *Tripping over patents: AIDS, access to treatment and the manufacturing of scarcity*. Unpublished Master's: University of Toronto.

Beyrer, C. 2003. Public health, human rights and the beneficience of states. *Human Rights Review*, October–December.

Bischoping, K. 1997. Responses to holocaust denial: A case study at the University of Michigan. *Contemporary Jewry*, 18.

Blandy, F. 2006. SA shows garlic and beetroot at AIDS conference. *Mail & Guardian Online*. <www.mg.co.za/article/2006-08-14-sa-shows-garlic-and-beetroot-at-aids-conference> accessed 25 August 2008.

Bond, P. 2001. *Against global apartheid: South Africa meets the World Bank, IMF and International Finance.* Lansdowne: UCT Press.

Bower, C.A. 1997. *The culture of denial: Why the environmental movement needs a strategy for reforming universities and public schools*. New York: SUNY Press.

Brown, D. 1997. US deaths from AIDS fall sharply better therapies get part of credit for drop. *Washington Post*, 28 February 1997.

Brulliard, K. 2009. Which Mrs Zuma will be South Africa's first lady? *Washington Post*, 9 May 2009. <www.washingtonpost.com/wp-dyn/content/article/2009/05/08/AR2009050803964.html> accessed 2 July 2009.

Buch, E. 2004. Equity in health care: Is the jury still out? In: C. Manganyi (ed.) *On becoming a democracy: Transition and transformation in South African society*. Pretoria: University of South Africa Press.

Burchell, J. 1990/91. AIDS and the law: Discrimination against the AIDS sufferer. *Businessman's Law*, 20.

Business Day, 10 September 2001.

Busse, P. 1995. Response of people with HIV and AIDS to representations of themselves. *AIDS Bulletin*, 4(1).

Butler, A. 2005. South Africa's HIV/AIDS Policy, 1994–2004: How can it be explained? *African Affairs*, 104(417).

Calms, G. 2008. South African resistance survey confirms that Clade C is more likely to develop multi-drug resistance mutation. *AIDS map news*. <www.aidsmap.com/en/news/2E39FB01-5534-444D-B693-72BDDD17BABC.asp?type=preview> accessed 2 June 2009.

Cameron, E. 1991. AIDS in employment – Facts, fantasies and fairness. *Employment Law*, 7(5).

Cameron, E. 1993a. Human rights, racism and AIDS: The new discrimination. *South African Journal on Human Rights*, 9.

Cameron, E. 1993b. Legal rights, human rights and AIDS: The first decade. *AIDS Analysis Africa*, 4(3).

Cameron, E. 2000. The deafening silence of AIDS. *Health and Human Rights*, 5(1).

Cameron, E. 2003. AIDS denial and holocaust denial – AIDS, justice and the courts in South Africa. *The South African Law Journal*, 120.

Cameron, E. and Swanson, E. 1992. Public health and human rights – The AIDS crisis in South Africa. *South African Journal on Human Rights*, 8.

Campbell, C., Foulis, C.A., Maimane, S. and Sibiya, Z. 2005. 'I have an evil child at my house': Stigma and HIV/AIDS management in a South African community. *American Journal of Public Health*, 95(5).

Chetty, M. 1993. Human rights, access to health care and AIDS. *South African Journal on Human Rights*, 9.

Chigwedere, P., Seage, G.R., Gruskin, S., Lee, T-H. and Essex, M. 2008. Estimating the lost benefits of antiretroviral drug use in South Africa. *J Acquir Immune DeficSyndr*, 49.

Cohan, J.A. 2002. 'I didn't know' and 'I was only doing my job': Has corporate governance careened out of control? A case study of Enron's information myopia. *Journal of Business Ethics*, 40.

Cohen, S. 1996. Government responses to human rights reports: Claims, denial and counterclaims. *Human Rights Quarterly*, 18.

Cohen, S. 2001. *States of denial: Knowing about atrocities and suffering*. Oxford: Blackwell.

Colvin, M. 1999. AIDS notification – Not a viable method of data gathering. *AIDS Bulletin*, 8(2).

Colvin, M. 2008. Impact of AIDS – The health care burden. In: S.S. Abdool Karim and Q. Abdool Karim (eds) *HIV/AIDS in South Africa*. Cambridge: Cambridge University Press.

Commerford, M.C., Orr, D.A., Gular, E., Reznikoff, M. and O'Dowd, M.A. 2006. Coping and psychological distress in women with HIV/AIDS. *Journal of Community Psychology*, 22(3).

Connor, E.M., Sperling, R.S., Gelber, R., Kiselev, P., Scott, G., O'Sullivan, M.J. et al. 1994. Reduction of maternal-infant transmission of Human Immunodeficiency Virus type 1 with zidovudine treatment. *The New England Journal of Medicine*, 331(18).

Corey, L., Wald, A., Celum, C.L. and Quinn, T. 2004. The effects of herpes simplex virus-2 on HIV-1 acquisition and transmission: A review of two overlapping epidemics. *J Acquir Immune DeficSyndr*, 35.

COSATU. 1991. Key policy issue papers and major resolutions from 4th National Congress, July 1991. *History in the Making*, 2(1).

Cowlin, J. 1999. Cheaper to manage HIV than to treat AIDS – The medscheme experience. *South African Medical Journal*, 89(1).

Crewe, M. 1996. How far has NACOSA plan been implemented? *AIDS Bulletin*, 5(2).

Crewe, M. 1999. Face of the future. *Siyaya*, 6 (Summer).

Crewe, M. 2000. How do we make sense of President Mbeki? *AIDS Analysis Africa*, 11(1).

Cullinan, K. 2008. MEC appoints task team to investigate 'racism' at Manguzi. *Health-e News Service*. <http://www.health-e.org.za/news/article.php?uid=20031946> accessed 3 January 2010.

Cullinan, K. and Thom, A. (eds) 2009. *The virus, vitamins and vegetables: The South African HIV/AIDS mystery*. Auckland Park: Jacana Media.

De Jager, F. 1991. VIGS: Die rol van die strafreg. *Journal of South African Law*, 2.

De Waal, A. 2003. How will HIV/AIDS transform African governance? *African Affairs*, 102(406).

De Waal, A. 2004. AIDS-related famine in Africa: Questioning assumptions and developing frameworks. In: N.K. Poku and A. Whiteside (eds) *The political economy of AIDS in Africa*. Aldershot: Ashgate.

De Waal, A. 2006. *AIDS and power: Why there is no political crisis yet*. London: Zed Books.

De Waal, A. and Whiteside, A. 2003. New variant famine: AIDS and food crisis in Southern Africa. *The Lancet*, 362.

Dorrington, R. and Johnson, L. 2002. Epidemiological and demographic. In: J. Gow and C. Desmond. *Impacts and interventions: The HIV and AIDS epidemic and the children of South Africa.* Pietermaritzburg: University of Natal Press.

Dorrington, R., Johnson, L., Bradshaw, D. and Daniel, T-J. 2006. *The demographic impact of HIV/AIDS in South Africa: National and provincial indicators for 2006*. The Center of Actuarial Research, the Burden of Disease Research Unit and the Actuarial Society of South Africa.

Draft Maputo Statement. 1991. Draft Maputo statement on HIV and AIDS in Southern Africa. *History in the Making*, 1(5).

Du Boisrouvray, A. 2000. Orphans and HIV: The second wave of the HIV epidemic. *Annals of the New York Academy of Sciences*, 918.

Du Plessis, M. 2000. The South African Employment Equity Act and HIV. *AIDS Analysis Africa*, 10(4).

Duesberg, P. 1991. AIDS epidemiology: Inconsistencies with Human Immunodeficiency Virus and with infectious disease. *Proceedings of the National Academy of Science*, 88.

Duesberg, P. and Rasnick, D. 1998. The AIDS dilemma: Drug diseases blamed on a passenger virus. *Genetica*, 104.

Dugger, C. 2008. Study cites toll of AIDS policy in South Africa. *The New York Times*, 26 November.

Dunkle, K.L., Jewkes, R.K., Brown, H.C., Gray, G.E., McIntryre, J.A. and Harlow, S.D. 2004. Transactional sex among women in Soweto, South Africa: Prevalence, risk factors and association with HIV infection. *Social Science and Medicine*, 59(8).

Editorial. 1987. AIDS virus research unit established. *MRC News*, 18(1).

Eichbaum, J. 1996. AIDS education: But who is being aided? *Scenaria*, 182.

Ekambaram, S. 1999. Health before profits. *Women's Health Project Newsletter*, 31.

Evian, C. 1995. AIDS, reconstruction and development and corporate response. *AIDS Analysis Africa*, 5(6).

Faris, S. 2004. Deadly denials as the nation struggles to accept the reality of AIDS. *Time International*, 163(16).

Fassin, D. 2007. *When bodies remember: Experiences and politics of AIDS in South Africa*. Berkeley: University of California Press.

Figueira, M. 2000. 'A' versus South African airways. *AIDS Legal Quarterly*, September.

Financial Mail, 14 June 1996.

Finansies en Tegniek, 13 September 1996.

Fischl, M.A., Richman, D.D., Grieco, M.H., Gottlieb, M.S., Volberding, P.A., Laskin, O.L., et al. 1987. The efficacy of azidothymidine (AZT) in the treatment of patients with AIDS and AIDS-related complex, a double-blind, placebo-controlled trial. *The New England Journal Of Medicine*, 317(4).

FitzSimons, D. 1990/91. AIDS and human rights. *AIDS Analysis Africa*, 2(4).
Fleming, A. 1994. A national AIDS plan for South Africa. *AIDS Analysis Africa*, 5(2).
Forman, L. 2003. Health legislation 1994–2003. In: P. Ujumba (ed) *South African Health Review 2003/04*. Johannesburg: Health Systems Trust.
Fourie, P. 2006. *The political management of HIV and AIDS in South Africa: One burden too many*? Houndmills: Palgrave Macmillan.
Fourie, P. and Schönteich, M. 2001. Africa's new security threat: HIV/AIDS and human security in Southern Africa. *African Security Review*, 10(4).
Fransen, L. 1998. HIV in developing countries. In: A. Whiteside (ed.) *Implications of AIDS for Demography and Policy in Southern Africa*. Pietermaritzburg: University of Natal Press.
Friedman, S. 1997. The revenge of the intellectuals: Policy research and dialogue in the new South Africa. *AIDS Bulletin*, 6(1/2).
Fröhlich, J. 2005. The impact of AIDS on the community. In: S.S. Abdool Karim and Q. Abdool Karim (eds) *HIV/AIDS in South Africa*. Cambridge: Cambridge University Press.
Furlong, P. and Ball, K. 2005. The more things change: AIDS and the state in South Africa, 1987–2003. In: A.S. Patterson (ed.) *The African state and the AIDS crisis*. Aldershot: Ashgate.
Galloway, M. 1996. Views from the regions. *AIDS Bulletin*, 5(2).
Galloway, M. 1999. Bringing together scientific rigour and public health needs. *AIDS Bulletin*, 8(1).
Galloway, M. 2000. South African National AIDS Council (SANAC) launched. *AIDS Bulletin*, 9(1).
Gaurie, V. and Lieberman, E.S. 2006. Boundary institutions and HIV/AIDS policy in Brazil and South Africa. *Studies in Comparative International Development*, 41(3).
Geffen, N. 2006. *Echoes of Lysenko: State-sponsored pseudo-science in South Africa*. CSSR Working Paper No. 149. Cape Town: Centre for Social Science Research.
Gevisser, M. 2007. *The dream deferred: Thabo Mbeki*. Johannesburg: Johnathan Ball Publishers.
Gill, P. 2006. *Body count: How they turned AIDS into a catastrophe*. Jeppestown: Jonathan Ball Publishers.
Gouws, E. and Abdool Karim, Q. 2008. HIV Infection in South Africa: The evolving pandemic. In: S.S. Abdool Karim and Q. Abdool Karim (eds) *HIV/AIDS in South Africa*. Cambridge: Cambridge University Press.
Government Gazette, R485, 23/4/99. Amendment to the regulations to communicable diseases and the notification of notifiable conditions.
Goyer, K. 2001. HIV and political instability in sub-Saharan Africa. *AIDS Analysis Africa*, 12(1).

Grundlingh, L. 1999. HIV and AIDS in South Africa: A case of failed responses because of stigmatisation, discrimination and morality, 1983–1994. *New Contree*, 46.

Grundlingh, L. 2001. Government responses to HIV/AIDS in South Africa as reported in the media, 1983–1994. *South African Historical Journal*, 45 (November).

Haarhoff, D. 2008. *Seven letters: HIV/AIDS stories from Namibian children.* Basel: BaslerAfrikaBibliographien.

Hadingham, J. 2000. Human security and Africa: Polemic opposites. *South African Journal of International Affairs*, 7(2).

Halperin, D.T. and Allen, A. 2001. Is poverty the root cause of African AIDS? *AIDS Analysis in Africa*, 11(4).

Halperin, D.T. and Epstein, H. 2007. Why is HIV prevalence so severe in Southern Africa? The role of multiple concurrent partnerships and lack of male circumcision: Implications for AIDS prevention. *The Southern African Journal of HIV Medicine*, March 2007.

Hambridge, M. 1990. Migrant labour and its impact on AIDS/HIV. *AIDS Analysis Africa*, 1(4).

Hatane, L. 1999. Ensuring political commitment and an expanded response to the HIV and AIDS epidemic. *AIDS Bulletin*, 8(2).

Hegarty, A. 2004. Truth, law and official denial: The case of Bloody Sunday. *Criminal Law Forum*, 15.

Heydt, H. 1992. HIV and AIDS policy statement: Practitioners corner. *The Journal of the Dental Association of South Africa*, 47(8).

Heywood, M. 1999. SADC moves towards making AIDS and HIV notifiable. *AIDS Analysis Africa*, 10(1).

Heywood, M. 2002. *From rhetoric to action – An evaluation of progress in relation to Priority Area 4: Human legal rights, HIV and AIDS National Plan.* Johannesburg: AIDS Law Project.

Heywood, M. 2004. The price of denial. *INTERFUND Development Update*, December 2004.

Heywood, M. 2007. *The end of politics? AIDS Law Project 18 Month Review: 2006 to 2007*. <http://www.alp.org.za/pdf/Publications/ALP%20Annual%20Reviews/ALP_2006-2007_Review.pdf> accessed 3 January 2010.

Heywood, M. 2008. The Achilles heel? The impact of HIV/AIDS on democracy in South Africa. In: S.S. Abdool Karim and Q. Abdool Karim (eds) *HIV/AIDS in South Africa*. Cambridge: Cambridge University Press.

Heywood, M. 2009. No easy walk to constitutional governance: The small matter of a health system. *AIDS Law Project 18-Month Review, 2007–08*. Johannesburg: AIDS Law Project.

Hickey, A. 2001. *Budgets and funding flows in the National Integrated Plan for HIV and AIDS.* Cape Town: IDASA.

Hickey, A., Ndlovu, N. and Guthrie, T. 2003. *Budgeting for HIV and AIDS in South Africa: Report on intergovernmental funding flows for an integrated response in the social sector.* Cape Town: IDASA.

Holmshaw, M. 1992. When will they ever learn? *Current AIDS Literature*, 5(5).

Hymes, K.B., Greene, J.B., Marcus, A., William, D.L., Cheung, T., Prose, N., Ballaro, H. and Canbestein, L. 1982. Kaposi's sarcoma in homosexual men: A report of eight cases. *The Lancet*, 2.

Jalusic, V. and Dedic, J. 2008. (The) Erasure – Mass human rights violation and denial of responsibility: The case of independent Slovenia. *Human Rights Review*, 9.

Jeter, J. 2000. South Africa's advances jeopardized by AIDS. *Washington Post*, 6 July 2000.

Jewkes, R., Sikweyiya, Y., Morrell, R. and Dunkle, K. 2009. *Understanding men's health and use of violence: Interface of rape and HIV in South Africa*. MRC Policy Brief, June 2009.

Jochelson, K., Mothibeli, M. and Leger, J. 1992. Human Immunodeficiency Virus and migrant labour in South Africa. *International Journal of Health Services*, 21(1).

Jones, P. and Koffeld, K. 2008. Governance matters for AIDS: But what about the politics? Lessons from South Africa and Uganda. In: M. Follér and H. Thörn (eds) *The politics of AIDS*. Houndmills: Palgrave Macmillan.

Joni, J. and Heywood, M. 2001. Error in judgement or failure by the judiciary to give clarity on the interpretation of the law? *AIDS Analysis Africa*, 12(3).

Joseph, C. 2002. HIV and AIDS and local government. *Occasional Paper*, 12.

Journal of Contemporary Roman-Dutch Law. 1992. Vonnisse. Vigs, boni mores en vertroulikheid. Johannesburg: Digma.

Kalichman, S.C. 2009. *Denying AIDS: Conspiracy theories, pseudoscience and human tragedy*. New York: Springer Science and Business Media.

Kalichman, S.C. and Simbayi, L.C. 2003. HIV testing attitudes, AIDS stigma and voluntary HIV counselling and testing in a black township in Cape Town, South Africa. *Sexually Transmitted Infections*, 79.

Kalichman, S.C., Simbayi, L.C., Kagee, A., Toefy, Y. and Jooste, S. 2006. Association of poverty, substance use and HIV transmission risk behaviors in three South African communities. *Social Science and Medicine*, 62.

Kallings, L.O. 2008. The first postmodern pandemic: 25 years of HIV/AIDS. *Journal of Internal Medicine*, 263.

Kaniki, A. 1999. Doing an information search. In: M. Terre Blanche and K. Durrheim (eds) *Research in Practice: Applied Methods for the Social Sciences*. Cape Town: UCT Press.

Karim, A. 1999. Making AIDS a notifiable disease – Is it an appropriate policy for South Africa? *South African Medical Journal*, 89(6).

Karim, Q. 1995. Government role in AIDS prevention and relationship with private sector. *AIDS Scan*, 7(3).

Karrim, Q. 2009. Calls for AIDS TRC. *Mail & Guardian Online*, 3 April 2009. <www.mg.co.za/article/2009-04-03-calls-calls-for-aids-trc> accessed 10 June 2009.

Kasper, T. 2002. Patents, pills and public policy: the pharmaceutical industry and international trade. In: K. Kelly, W. Parker and S. Gelby (eds) *HIV and AIDS, economics and governance in South Africa: Key issues in understanding response*. Johannesburg: CADRE.

Kher, U. 2003. July 27, 1982: A name for the plague. *Time Magazine*, 31 March. <http://www.time.com/time/80days/820727.html> accessed 10 June 2009.

Killian, B. 2004. Risk and resilience. In: Pharoah, R. (ed.) *A generation at risk? HIV/AIDS, vulnerable children and security in Southern Africa*. Monograph 109, December. Pretoria: Institute for Security Studies.

Kirby, M. 1993a. AIDS and the law. *South African Journal on Human Rights*, 9.

Kirby, M. 1993b. Life's dominion – Closing reflections. *South African Journal on Human Rights*, 9.

Kitching, G. 1996. Sal 'Sarafina' VIGS oorleef? *Insig* (April).

Klouda, T. 1994. It's called 'Fiddling while Rome burns'. *AIDS Analysis Africa*, 5(2).

Kometsi, K. 2004. *(Un)real: AIDS review 2004*. Pretoria: University of Pretoria.

Kopelman, L.M. 2005. If HIV/AIDS is punishment, who is bad? In: A.A. Van Niekerk and L.M. Kopelman (eds) *Ethics and AIDS in Africa: The challenge to our thinking*. Claremont: David Philip.

Labour Bulletin. 1989. Briefings: Mineworkers tackle health and safety. *Labour Bulletin*, 14(4).

Lagarde, E., Dirk, T., Puren, A., Reathe, R-T. and Bertran, A. 2003. Acceptability of male circumcision as a tool for preventing HIV infection in a highly infected community in South Afric. *AIDS*, 17.

Lasson, K. 2007. Defending truth: Legal and psychological aspects of holocaust denial. *Current Psychology*, 26.

Leclerc-Madlala, S. 2003. Transactional sex and the pursuit of modernity. *Social Dynamics*, 29(2).

Leclerc-Madlala, S. 2008. *Intergenerational/age-disparate sex*. Technical meeting on young women in HIV hyper-endemic countries of Southern Africa. Geneva: UNAIDS.

Leech, B. 1993. The right of the HIV-positive patient to medical care: An analysis of the costs of providing medical treatment. *South African Journal on Human Rights*, 9.

Leech, B. 1994. The Charter of Rights on AIDS and HIV: Panacea or chimera. *South African Public Law*, 9(2).

Lekotjolo, N. 2009. Charge Mbeki and Manto with genocide. *The Sunday Times*, 8 November.

Lemey, P., Pybus, O.G., Wang, B., Saksena, N.K., Salemi, M. and Vandamme, A-M. 2003. Tracing the origin and history of the HIV-2 epidemic. *PNAS*, 100(11).

Lewis, S. 2006. Remarks by Stephen Lewis, UN Special Envoy for HIV/AIDS in Africa, to the closing session of the XVI International AIDS Conference,

Toronto, Canada. *Kaisernetwork*. <www.kaisernetwork.org/health_cast/uploaded_files/Lewis%20 Closing%20Speech.pdf> accessed 17 August 2008.

Lodge, T. 2002. *Politics in South Africa: From Mandela to Mbeki*. Indiana: Indiana University Press.

Lombard, A. 2008. Desperate doctors. *Health-e News Service*. <http://www.health-e.org.za/news/article.php?uid=20032085> accessed 3 January 2010.

Lurie, M. 2000. Migration and AIDS in South Africa: A review. *South African Journal of Science*, 96(6).

Lush, L. and Makoala, S. 1999. Implementing policies to integrate HIV/STD services with primary health care in Northern Province, South Africa. *Women's Health Project Newsletter*, 31.

Mabogoane, M. 2008. Mbeki's legacy not his alone. *Mail & Guardian*, 8 October.

Mail & Guardian, 26 October 2000.

Mail & Guardian, 28 September 2000.

Makgoba, M. 2001. HIV: The greatest threat to the African Renaissance. *MRC News*, 32(4).

Manning, R. 2001. *Noble intentions, harsh realities: The politics of AIDS policy in South Africa.* Unpublished Thesis: Woodrow Wilson School of Public and International Affairs.

Marais, H. 1998. *South Africa: Limits to change: The political economy of transformation.* Cape Town: UCT Press.

Marais, H. 2000. *To the edge: AIDS review 2000*. Pretoria: Centre for the Study of AIDS.

Marais, H. 2005. *Buckling: The impact of AIDS in South Africa 2005*. Pretoria: Centre for the Study of AIDS.

Markowitz, G.E. and Rosner, D. 2003. *Deceit and denial: The deadly politics of industrial pollution.* Berkeley: University of California Press.

Marks, S. 2008. The burdens of the past. In: A. Ndinga-Muvumba and R. Pharoah (eds) *HIV/AIDS and society in South Africa*. Scottsville: University of Kwa-Zulu Natal Press.

Mattes, R. and Manning, R. 2004. The impact of HIV/AIDS on democracy in Southern Africa: What do we know, what do we need to know and why? In: N.K. Poku and A. Whiteside (eds) *The political economy of AIDS in Africa.* Aldershot: Ashgate.

Mbali, M. 2003. HIV and AIDS policy-making in post-apartheid South Africa. In: J. Daniel, A. Habib and R. Southal (eds) *State of the Nation: South Africa 2003–2004.* Cape Town: HSRC Press.

Mbeki, T. 1999. The South African declaration on AIDS. *The South African Dental Journal*, 54(12).

Mbeki, T. 2000. Mbeki's letter to world leaders on AIDS in Africa. *The Memory Hole*. <www.floonet.net/articles/mbeki.shtml> accessed 10 June 2009.

Mbeki, T. 2001. Address by President Thabo Mbeki, at the inaugural ZK Matthews Memorial Lecture, University of Fort Hare, 12 October 2001. *Government*

Speeches. <www.info.gov.za/speeches/2001/011016442p1001.htm> accessed 10 June 2009.

Mbeki, T. and Leon, T. 2000. Correspondence between Thabo Mbeki and Tony Leon. Originally published in the Sunday Times. *Virusmyth.com*. <http://www.virusmyth.com/aids/news/letmbeki.htm> accessed 4 June 2009.

MCC. 2009. Medicines Control Council – Home Page. *MCC*. <http://www.mccza.com/main.asp> accessed 15 May 2009.

McCutchan, F.E. 2000. Understanding the genetic diversity of HIV-1. *AIDS*, 2000(14).

McGregor, L. 2009. Garlic, olive oil, lemons and beetroot. In: K. Culminant and A. Thom (eds) *The virus, vitamins and vegetables: The South African HIV/AIDS mystery*. Auckland Park: Jacana Media.

McInnes, C. 2006. HIV/AIDS and security. *International Affairs*, 82(2).

McKerrow, N. 2002. Treatment of HIV and AIDS and related illnesses. In: J. Gow and C. Desmond (eds) *Impacts and interventions: The HIV and AIDS epidemic and the children of South Africa*. Pietermaritzburg: University of Natal Press.

McKerrow, N. 2003. The South African response to the HIV and AIDS epidemic: An input paper to the report on the elimination of poverty and inequality in South Africa.

McKinnon, C. 2007. Should we tolerate holocaust denial? *Res Publica*, 13.

McPherson, M.F., Hoover, D. and Snodgrass, D.R. 2000. *The impact on economic growth in Africa of rising costs and labor productivity losses associated with HIV/AIDS*. CAER II Discussion Paper No. 79. Cambridge: Harvard Institute for International Development.

MMWR. 1981a. Pneumocystis pneymonia – Los Angeles. *Morbidity and Mortality Weekly Report*, June 5, 30(21).

MMWR. 1981b. Kaposi's Sarcoma and pneumocystis pneumonia among homosexual men – New York City and California. *Morbidity and Mortality Weekly Report*, July 4, 31(4).

MMWR. 1983. Epidemiologic notes and reports on immunodeficiency among female sexual partners of males with Acquired Immune Deficiency Syndrome (AIDS) – New York. *Morbidity and Mortality Weekly Report*, March 4, 32(8).

Monasch, R. and Snoad, N. 2003. *The situation of orphans in a region affected by HIV/AIDS*. Papcr presented at the scientific meeting on empirical evidence for the demographic and socio-economic impact of AIDS, hosted by HEARD. 26–28 March 2003, Durban.

Moodie, J. 1988. Serology of AIDS. *South African Journal of Continuing Medical Education*, 6(3).

Morris, M. and Kretzschmar, M. 1997. Concurrent partnerships and the spread of HIV. *AIDS*, 11.

Motobele, T. and Heywood, M. 2001. South Africa's constitutional court declares pre-employment testing a human rights violation. *AIDS Analysis Africa*, 11(4).

Murphy, V. 2003. Mbeki stirs up AIDS controversy. *BBC News*. <http://news.bbc.co.uk/2/hi/africa/3143850.stm> accessed 4 June 2008.

Myburgh, J. 2007. The Virodene affair. *Politicsweb*. <www.politicsweb.co.za/politicsweb/view/politicsweb/en/page71619?oid=83156&sn=Detail> accessed 24 May 2009.

National Institute of Allergy and Infectious Diseases. 2003. The evidence that HIV causes AIDS. *National Institutes of Health: US Department of Health and Human Services*. <www.niaid.nih.gov/factsheets/evidhiv.htm> accessed 2 June 2008.

Nattrass, N. 2004. *The moral economy of AIDS in South Africa*. Cambridge: Cambridge University Press.

Nattrass, N. 2005. Rolling out antiretroviral treatment in South Africa: Economic and ethical challenges. In: A.A. Van Niekerk and L.M. Kopelman (eds) *Ethics and AIDS in Africa: The challenge to our thinking*. Claremont: David Philip.

Nattrass, N. 2007. *Mortal combat: AIDS denialism and the struggle for antiretrovirals in South Africa*. Scottsville: University of KwaZulu-Natal Press.

Ndinga-Muvumba, A. and Scanlon, H. 2006. *AIDS and society in South Africa: Building a community of practice*. Cape Town: Centre for Conflict Resolution.

Nelson, R. 2006. AIDS treatment enters its 25th year. *The Lancet*, 6.

Nepal, B. 2007. AIDS denial in Asia: Dimensions and roots. *Health Policy*, 84.

News24, 18 January 2005.

News24, 24 January 2005.

Ngonyama, S. 2000. A virus cannot cause a syndrome. *Business Day*, 4 October.

Ngwena, C. and Pelser, A. 2001 Strengthening local government and civic responses to the HIV/AIDS epidemic: A study for the Ford Foundation. Working Paper: Centre for Health Systems Research and Development, University of the Free State.

Oosthuizen, I. 1994. The management of AIDS in South African schools. *Koers: Bulletin for Christian Scholarship*, 59(2).

Papathanasopoulos, M.A., Hunt, G.M. and Thiemessen, C.T. 2003. Evolution and diversity of HIV-1 in Africa: A review. *Virus Genes*, 2003(26).

Parker, W. 1996. A national media campaign: Who makes the decisions and what is really needed? *AIDS Bulletin*, 5(2).

Parker, W., Makhubele, B., Ntlabati, P. and Connolly, C. 2007. *Concurrent sexual partnerships amongst young adults in South Africa: Challenges for HIV prevention communication*. Grahamstown: CADRE.

Pear, R. 1985. AIDS blood test to be available in 2 to 6 weeks. *The New York Times*, 3 March.

Peltzer, K. 2008. The public education sector and HIV/AIDS. In: N. Ndinga-Muvumba and R. Pharoah (eds) *HIV/AIDS and society in South Africa*. Scottsville: University of Kwa-Zulu Natal Press.

Pettifor, A.E., Rees, H.V., Kleinschmidt, I., Steffenson, A.E., MacPhail, C., Hlongwa-Madikisela, L., Vermaak, K. and Padian, N.C. 2005. Young people's sexual health in South Africa: HIV prevalence and sexual behaviors from a nationally representative household survey. *AIDS*, 19(14).

Phila. 1996. The Sarafina II controversy. *Phila Legislative Update*, 3.

Poku, N.K. 2004. Confronting AIDS with debt: Africa's silent crisis. In: N.K. Poku and A. Whiteside (eds) *The political economy of AIDS in Africa*. Aldershot: Ashgate.

Poku, N.K. and Whiteside, A. 2006. 25 Years of living with HIV/AIDS: Challenges and prospects. *International Affairs*, 82(2).

Power, R., Koopman, C., Volk, J., Israelski, D.M., Stone, L., Chesney, M.A. and Spiegel, D. 2003. Social support, substance use and denial in relationship to antiretroviral treatment adherence among HIV-infected persons. *AIDS Patient Care and STDs*, 17(5).

Power, S. 2003. The AIDS rebel letter from South Africa. *The New Yorker*, 79(12).

Price, M. and Van den Heever, A. 1994. The Reconstruction and development programme and health. *Southern African Journal of Epidemiology and Infection*, 9(2).

Priority Press. 1995. *Update on combination antiretroviral therapy: Results of the Delta study*. The Fifth European Conference on clinical aspects and treatment of HIV Infection, Copenhagen Denmark, 26–29 September 1995. <www.mednet.ca/html/ppaids07.htm> accessed 4 March 2009.

Radebe, J. 2007. *Speech by the acting Minister of Health at the National Consultative Conference on HIV and AIDS*, Department of Health, 14 March 2007.

Raphaely, C. 1989. Frightening figures. *Finance Week*, 42(5).

Ras, G.J., Simson, I.W., Anderson, R., Prozesky, O.W. and Hamersma, T. 1983. Acquired Immunodeficiency Syndrome: A report of 2 South African cases. *South African Medical Journal*, 64.

Richter, L. 2004. The impact of HIV/AIDS on the development of children. In: R. Pharoah (ed.) *A generation at risk? HIV/AIDS, vulnerable children and security in Southern Africa*. Monograph 109. December. Pretoria: Institute for Security Studies.

Roberts, R.S. 2007. *Fit to govern: The native intelligence of Thabo Mbeki*. Johannesburg: STE Publishers.

Rödlach, A. 2006. *Witches, westerners and HIV: AIDS and cultures of blame in Africa*. Walnut Creek: Left Coast Press.

Sadie, Y. and Van Aardt, M. 1992. Vigs-Politiek in Suid Afrika: 1987–1992. *Politikon*, 19(3).

Sadie, Y., Van Aardt, M. and Verwey, S. 1994. Public policy formulation and implementation as political communication: The case of AIDS in South Africa. *Communitas: Journal for Community Communication*, 1.

SAPA, 4 April 2001.

SAPA, 14 November 2001.

Sarkin, J. 1993. Health. *South African Human Rights Yearbook 1994*, 5.

Scheider, M. and Moodie, M. 2002. *The destabilising impacts of HIV/AIDS*. Washington, DC: Center for Strategic and International Studies.

Schneider, H. 1998. *The politics behind AIDS: The case of South Africa*. Johannesburg: Centre for Health Policy.

Schneider, H. 2001. *The AIDS impasse in South Africa as a struggle for symbolic power*. Johannesburg: Centre for Health Policy.

Schneider, H. 2002. On the fault-line: The politics of AIDS policy in contemporary South Africa. *African Studies*, 61(1).

Schneider, H. and Fassin, D. 2002. Denial and defiance: A socio-political analysis of AIDS in South Africa. *AIDS*, 16(4).

Schneider, H. and McIntyre, J. 1994. Is the 1993/94 AIDS programme budget adequate? *AIDS Scan*, 6(2).

Schneider, H. and Stein, J. 2001. Implementing AIDS policy in post-apartheid South Africa. *Social Science and Medicine*, 52.

Schrire, R. 2001. The realities of opposition in South Africa: Legitimacy, strategies and consequences. *Democratization*, 8(1).

Serpa, E. 2002. AIDS in Africa: The social-cultural roots of a disease. *Africa Insight*, 32(3).

Serwadda, D., Mugerwa, R.D., Sewankambo, N.K., Lwegaba, A., Carswell, J.W., Kirya, G.B., Bayley, A.C,, Tedder, R.S., Weiss, R.A., Downing, R.G., Clayden, S.A. and Dalgleish, A.G. 1985. Slim disease: A new disease in Uganda and its association with HTLV-III Infection. *The Lancet*, 2(8460).

Setiloane, M. 1991. AIDS in South Africa: Some issues and considerations. *Social Work Practice*.

Sher, R. 1989. HIV infection in South Africa, 1982–1988: A review. *South African Medical Journal*, 76(Oct).

Sher, R. 1990. Women and HIV and AIDS. *AIDS Scan*, 2(4).

Sherr, L., Christie, G., Sher, R. and Mets, J. 1989. Evaluation of the effectiveness of AIDS training and information courses in South Africa. *AIDS Scan*, 2.

Singh, J. 2005. The impact on ethics. In: S.S. Abdool Karim and Q. Abdool Karim (eds) *HIV/AIDS in South Africa*. Cambridge: Cambridge University Press.

Sishana, O. 2008. *HIV/AIDS and Society*. Paper prepared for the presidency as part of the fifteen year review process. <www.thepresidency.gov.za/docs/reports/15year_review/ social/hiv_aids.pdf> accessed 5 June 2009.

Sitze, A. 2004. Denialism. *South Atlantic Quarterly*, 103(4).

Smart, R. 2002. Preventing transmission of HIV. In: J. Gow and C. Desmond. *impacts and interventions: The HIV and AIDS epidemic and the children of South Africa*. Pietermaritzburg: University of Natal Press.

Smith, A. 1999. Notification of HIV and AIDS. *AIDS Bulletin* (July).

Sontag, S. 2002. *Illness as metaphor and AIDS and its metaphors*. London: Penguin Group.

Southern African Practice Management. 1992. First SA court ruling on doctor's duty of confidentiality towards patient with AIDS. *Southern African Practice Management*, 13(1).

Sparks, A. 2003. *Beyond the miracle: Inside the new South Africa.* London: Profile Books.

Specter, M. 2007. The denialists: The dangerous attacks on the consensus about HIV and AIDS. *The New Yorker*, March 12.

Spencer, D. 1995. The management of South Africa's HIV infected: What are the challenges? *South African Journal of Epidemiology and Infection*, 10(2).

Statistics SA. 2008. *Mid-year population estimates 2008: Statistical release P0302*. Pretoria: Statistics SA.

Stein, J. 2003. *Sorrow makes children of us all: A literature review on the psycho-social impact of HIV/AIDS on children*. Working Paper 47. Cape Town: Centre for Social Science Research.

Steinberg, M. 1993. The national AIDS research programme of the MRC. *AIDS Analysis Africa*, 4(2).

Stephen, J. 2009. 'Saints and sinners': The Treatment Action Campaign. In: K. Cullinan and A. Thom (eds) *The virus, vitamins and vegetables: The South African HIV/AIDS mystery*. Auckland Park: Jacana Media.

Strachan, K. 1995. The month in review. *HST Update*, 5.

Strachan, K. 1996. The current health budget: Who gets what? *South African Family Practice*, 17(7).

Strand, P., Matlosa, K., Strode, A. and Chirambo, K. 2004. *HIV/AIDS and democratic governance in South Africa: Illustrating the impact on electoral processes*. Pretoria: Institute for Democracy in South Africa (IDASA).

Strategic Plan. 2000. *HIV and AIDS/STD Strategic Plan for South Africa 2000–2005*.

Strauss, S. 1988. Legal issues concerning AIDS: An outline. *South African Practice Management*, 9(1).

Streek, B. and Forrest, D. 2001. Mbeki in bizarre AIDS outburst. *Mail & Guardian Online*, 26 October 2001. <http://www.mg.co.za> accessed 25 August 2008.

Strode, A. 1994. Patients are people with rights. *Positive Outlook*, 1(3).

Strode, A. and Grant, K. 2004. *Understanding the institutional dynamics of South Africa's response to HIV and AIDS pandemic.* Pretoria: IDASA.

Taylor, G. 1994. Employers still cautious. *AIDS Analysis Africa*, 5(1).

The Body. 2009. Inspiring stories of people affected by HIV/AIDS. *The Body.com*. <http://www.thebody.com/index/inspire.html> accessed 25 May, 2009.

The Guardian, 6 November 2007.

The Lancet. 2005. South Africa needs to face the truth about HIV mortality. *The Lancet*, 365(9459).

The Lancet. 2006. Editorial: South Africa needs and HIV truth and reconciliation commission. *The Lancet*, 367.

The Perth Group. 2008. The AIDS debate. *The Perth Group*. <www.theperthgroup.com> accessed 3 July 2008.

The Star, 4 March 2003.

Thom, A. 2009. The curious tale of the vitamin seller. In: K. Cullinan and A. Thom (eds) *The virus, vitamins and vegetables: The South African HIV/AIDS mystery*. Auckland Park: Jacana Media.

Treichler, P. 1999. *How to have theory in an epidemic: Cultural chronicles of AIDS*. London: Duke University Press.

Trengove-Jones, T. 2001. *Who cares? AIDS Review 2001*. Pretoria: University of Pretoria.

Ulin, P. 1992. African women and AIDS: Negotiating behavioural change. *AIDS Scan*, 4(3).

UNAIDS. 2004. *Epidemiological fact sheets on HIV/AIDS and sexually transmitted infections – South Africa*. Geneva: UNAIDS.

UNAIDS. 2006. *2006 Report on the global AIDS epidemic*. Geneva: UNAIDS.

UNAIDS. 2007. *AIDS epidemic update: 2007 December*. Geneva: UNAIDS.

UNAIDS. 2008. *2008 Report on the global AIDS epidemic*. Geneva: UNAIDS.

UNAIDS. 2009. *Key populations: Women and girls*, Joint United Nations Programme on HIV/AIDS. Geneva: UNAIDS. <www.unaids.org/en/PolicyAndPractice/KeyPopulations/Women Girls/default.asp> accessed 12 June 2009.

UNDP. 2004. *Thailand's response to HIV/AIDS: Progress and challenges*. UNDP.

United Nations Department of Economic and Social Affairs. 2004. New York: United Nations Publication.

Van Ammers, P. 1990. Human Immunodeficiency Virus in obstetrics. *South African Journal of Continuing Medical Education*, 8(3).

Van der Linde, I. 1999. The costing of HIV and AIDS – Without a clue? *AIDS Scan*, 11(1).

Van der Vliet, V. 2001. AIDS: Losing 'the new struggle?' *Daedalus*, 130(1).

Van der Vliet, V. 2004a. Dealing with AIDS: A work in progress. *Focus*, 34.

Van der Vliet, V. 2004b. South Africa divided against AIDS: A crisis of leadership. In: K. Kauffman and D. Lindauer (eds) *AIDS and South Africa: The social expression of a pandemic*. Basingstoke: Macmillan.

Van Dijk, T.A. 1992. Discourse and the denial of racism. *Discourse and Society*, 3.

Van Heuverswyn, F., Li, Y., Neel, C., Bailes, E., Keele, B.F., Liu, W., Takehisa, J., Santiago, M.L., Bibollet-Ruche, F., Chen, Y., Wain, L.V., Liegeois, F., Loul, S., Mpoudi Ngole, E., Bienvenue, Y., Delaporte, E., Brookfield, J.F.Y., Sharp, P.M., Shaw, G.M., Peeters, M. and Hahn, B.H. 2006. Chimpanzee reservoirs of pandemic and nonpandemic HIV-1. *Science*, 313.

Van Niekerk, A.A. 2001. Moral and social complexities of AIDS in Africa. *Journal of Medicine and Philosophy*, 27(2).

Van Wyk, C. 1992. Vigs en bloedoortrappings: Enkele regaspekte. *De Jure*, 1.

Viljoen, F. 1993. Verligting of verlustiging: Regshervorming in 'n tyd van Vigs. *The South African Law Journal*, 110.

Von Mollendorff, T. 2009. Daring to care: A doctor's persecution in Mpumalanga. In: K. Cullinan and A. Thom (eds) *The virus, vitamins and vegetables: The South African HIV/AIDS mystery*. Auckland Park: Jacana Media.

Walker, L., Reid, G. and Cornell, M. 2004. *Waiting to happen: HIV and AIDS in South Africa*. Colorado: Lynne Rienner Publishers.

Wang, J. 2008. AIDS denialism and 'The humanisation of the African'. *Race and Class*, 49(1).

Washington Post, 14 July 2000.

Washington Post, 15 March 2001.

Washington Post, 29 April 2004.

Wawer, M.J., Makumbi, F., Kgigozi, G., Serwadda, D., Watya, S., Nalugoda, F., Buwembo, D., Ssempijja, V., Kiwanuka, N., Moulton, L.H., Sewankambo, N.K., Reynolds, S.J., Quinn, T.C., Opendi, P., Iga, B., Ridzon, R., Laeyendecker, O. and Gray, R.H. 2009. Circumcision in HIV-infected mean and its effect on HIV transimission to female partners in Rakai, Uganda: A randomised controlled trial. *The Lancet*, 374(9685).

Weiss, H.A., Quigley, M.A. and Hayes, R.J. 2000. Male circumcision and risk of HIV infection in sub-Saharan Africa: A systematic review and meta-analysis. *AIDS*, 14.

Welch, M. 2003. Trampling human rights in the War on Terror: Implications to the sociology of denial. *Critical Criminology*, 12.

Whiteside, A. 1991. Lessons from Africa. *AIDS Analysis Africa*, 1(5).

Whiteside, A. 1993. AIDS in South Africa: The first ten years. *AIDS Bulletin*, 4(2).

Whiteside, A. 1998. Policymakers' and planners' needs in projecting the epidemic. In: A. Whiteside (ed.) *Implications of AIDS for demography and policy in Southern Africa.* Pietermaritzburg: University of Natal Press.

Whiteside, A. 2004. Responding to AIDS in crisis situations. In: N.K. Poku and A. Whiteside (eds) *The political economy of AIDS in Africa.* Aldershot: Ashgate.

Whiteside, A. 2005. The economic impact of AIDS. In: S.S. Abdool Karim and Q. Abdool Karim (eds) *HIV/AIDS in South Africa.* Cambridge: Cambridge University Press.

Whiteside, A. 2006. HIV/AIDS and development: Failures of vision and imagination. *Journal of International Affairs*, 82(2).

Whiteside, A. and Sunter, C. 2000. *AIDS: The challenge for South Africa.* Cape Town: Human and Rousseau/Tafelberg.

Whiteside, A., Barnett, T., George, G. and Van Niekerk, A.A. 2005. Through a glass, darkly: data and uncertainty in the AIDS debate. In: A.A. Van Niekerk and L.M. Kopelman (eds) *Ethics and AIDS in Africa: The challenge to our thinking*. Claremont: David Philip.

Whiteside, A., Mattes, R., Willian, S. and Manning, R. 2004. What people really believe about HIV/AIDS in Southern Africa. In: N.K. Poku and A. Whiteside (eds) *The political economy of AIDS in Africa*. Aldershot: Ashgate.

WHO. 2008. *Towards universal access: Scaling up priority HIV/AIDS interventions in the health sector: Progress report 2008*. Geneva: World Health Organisation.

Wilkinson, D., Floyd, K. and Gilks, C. 1999. A national programme to reduce mother-to-child HIV transmission is potentially cost saving. *AIDS Bulletin*, 8(1).

Winsbury, P. 1992. Where the AIDS war can be won. *AIDS Analysis Africa*, 2(5).

World Bank. 1999. *World development report: Knowledge for development*. Oxford: Oxford University Press.

Worobey, M., Gemmel, M., Teuwen, D.E., Haselkorn, T., Kuntsman, K., Bunce, M., Muyembe, J.-J., Kabongo, J-M.M., Kalengayi, R.M., Van Marck, E., Thomas, M., Gilbert, P. and Wolinsky, S.M. 2008. Direct evidence of extensive diversity of HIV-1 in Kinshasa by 1960. *Nature*, 455.

Yach, D. 1992. Development and health: The need for integrated approaches in South Africa. *Development Southern Africa*, 9(1).

Youde, J.R. 2007. *AIDS, South Africa and the politics of knowledge*. Aldershot: Ashgate.

Zapiro, 2005. Zapiro for January 4, 2005. *Mail & Guardian Online*. <http://www.mg.co.za/zapiro/fullcartoon/816> accessed 10 June 2009.

Zerouali, A. 1999. Government responses to the Massacres. In: Y. Bedjaoui, A. Aroua and M. Ait-Larbi (eds) *An inquiry into the Algerian massacres*. Geneva: Hoggar Books.

Zuma, B. 1996. Cross-Cultural counselling. *Positive Outlook*, 3(4).

Index

For Product Safety Concerns and Information please contact our EU representative GPSR@taylorandfrancis.com Taylor & Francis Verlag GmbH, Kaufingerstraße 24, 80331 München, Germany

Batch number: 10725802

Printed by Printforce, the Netherlands